# KETO MEAL PREP

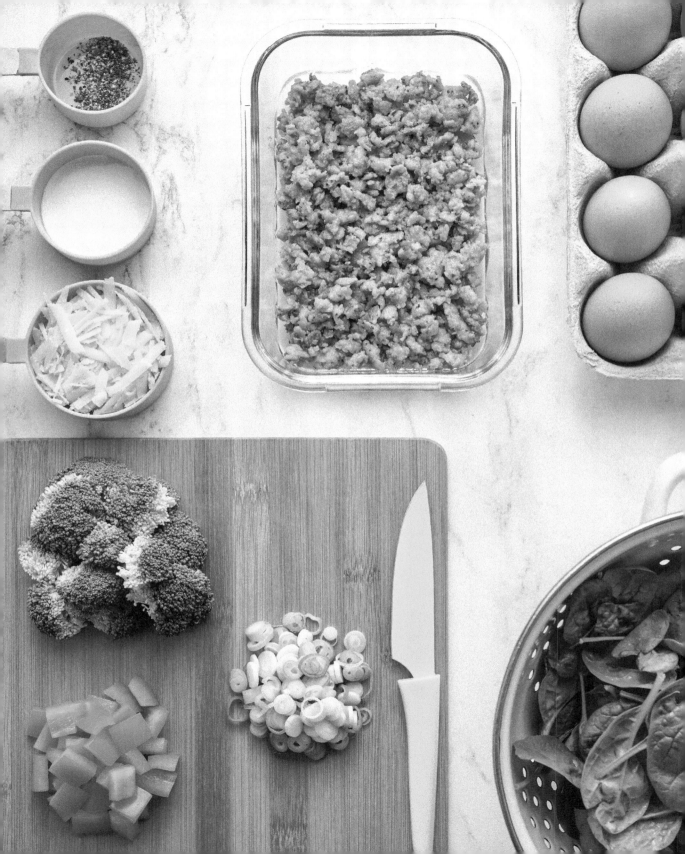

# keto
# MEAL
# PREP

**Lose Weight, Save Time,
and Feel Your Best
on the Ketogenic Diet**

## LIZ WILLIAMS

Photography by Darren Muir

ROCKRIDGE
PRESS

## A labor of love for the ketogenic community.

Interior Designer: Chris Fong
Cover Designer: Will Mack
Editor: Stacy Wagner-Kinnear
Production Editor: Andrew Yackira
Photography: Darren Muir

ISBN: Print 978-1-64152-247-2 | eBook 978-1-64152-248-9

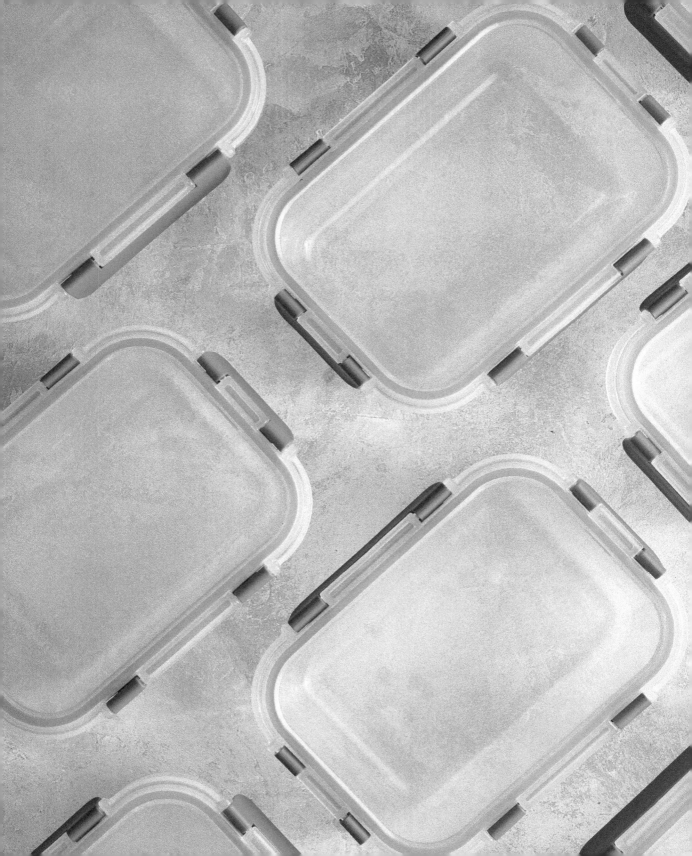

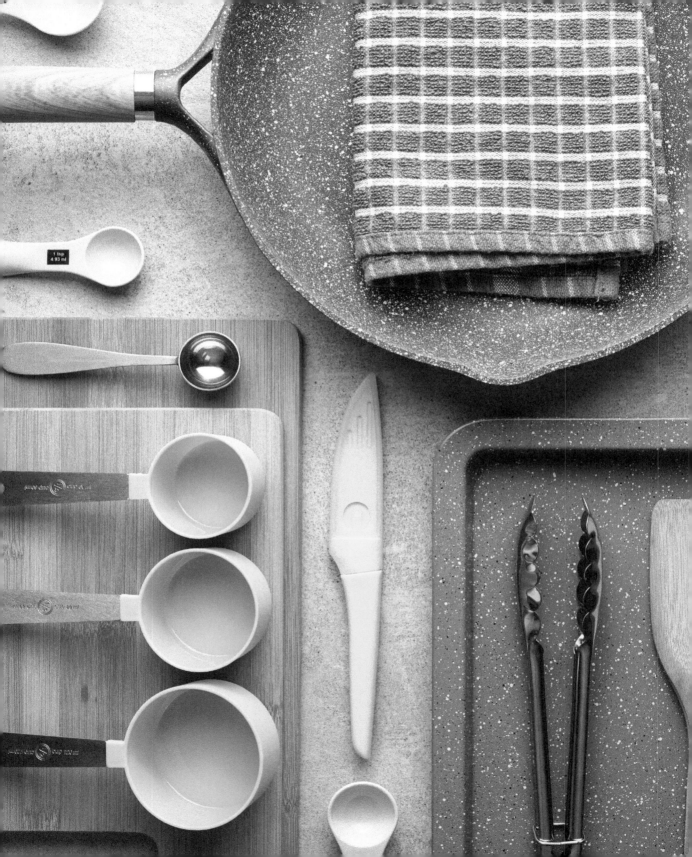

# Contents

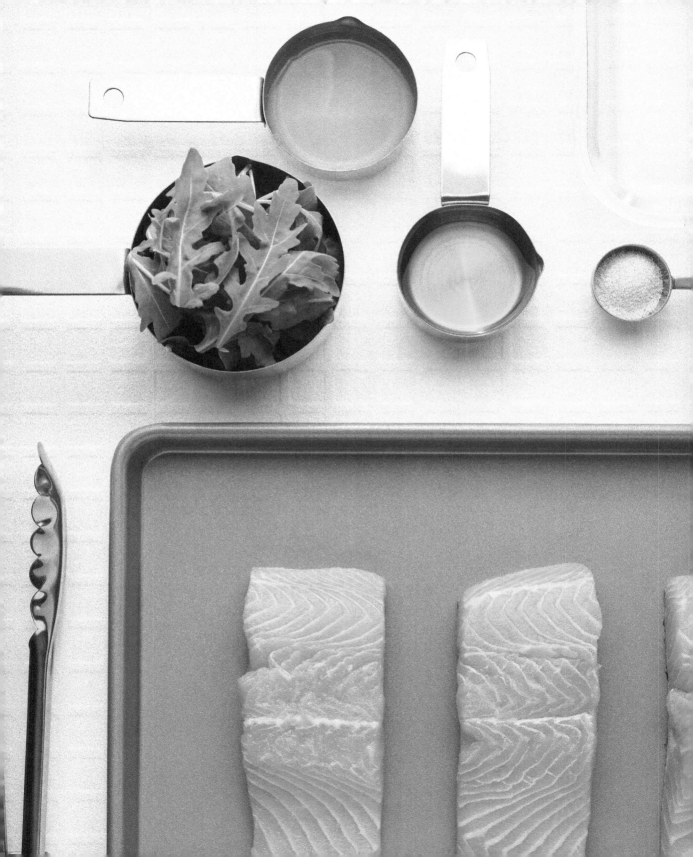

# Introduction

When I began my fitness journey six years ago, my husband worked as a personal trainer and I was working at a hospital. We decided to commit to our nutrition rather than just our gym time. That's when our bodies really started to change and when we dialed in our nutrition and were consistent with our time in the gym.

Back then, our meal preps consisted of a lot of brown rice, lean protein, egg whites, sweet potatoes, and bland vegetables. We definitely saw results but not as many benefits as we did when we turned to the ketogenic diet.

I am so thankful we started keto when we did and meal prep became something we practiced together each week. It is a habit we still practice today. The biggest difference between our previous diet and keto is that now we eat a lot of healthy fats and satiating foods. Some benefits to living keto that we've experienced are mental clarity, strengthened immunity, sustainable lean muscle mass, effortless fasting, and being able to eat foods we truly enjoy.

When I started my ketogenic journey, I couldn't believe how many options I had and how creative I could be in the kitchen. It was so freeing after living the typical bodybuilder's program. One thing that was hard about starting keto was all the contradicting information out there. But keto doesn't need to be difficult; it truly is as simple as including a fat, a protein, and a green vegetable in your meals. Don't make it more complicated than that.

I hope you will find tools within these pages that will make your daily life easier and less stressful. I know making the time to plan and prep ahead will save you money, time, and your health.

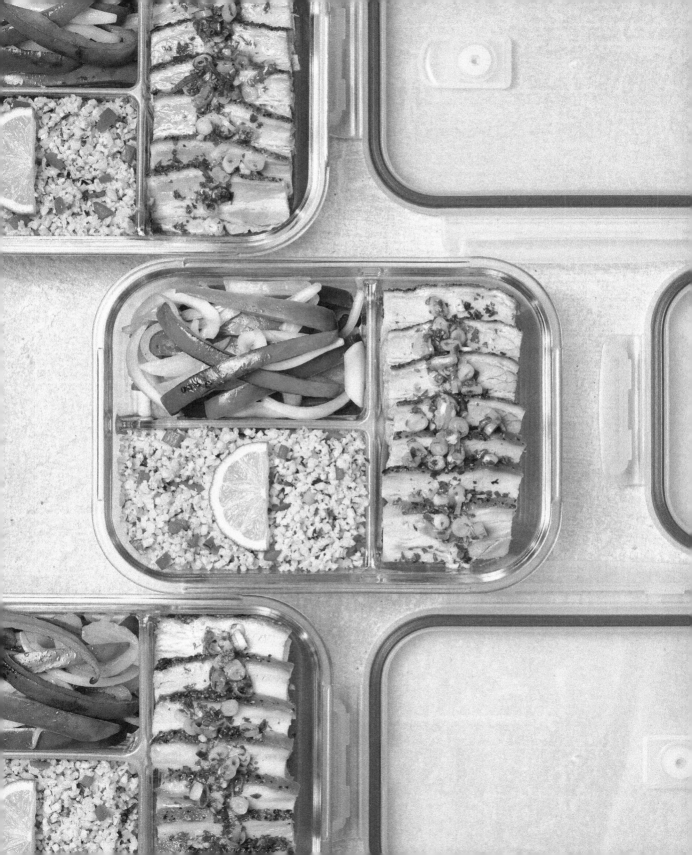

# PART ONE

# READY-TO-GO KETO

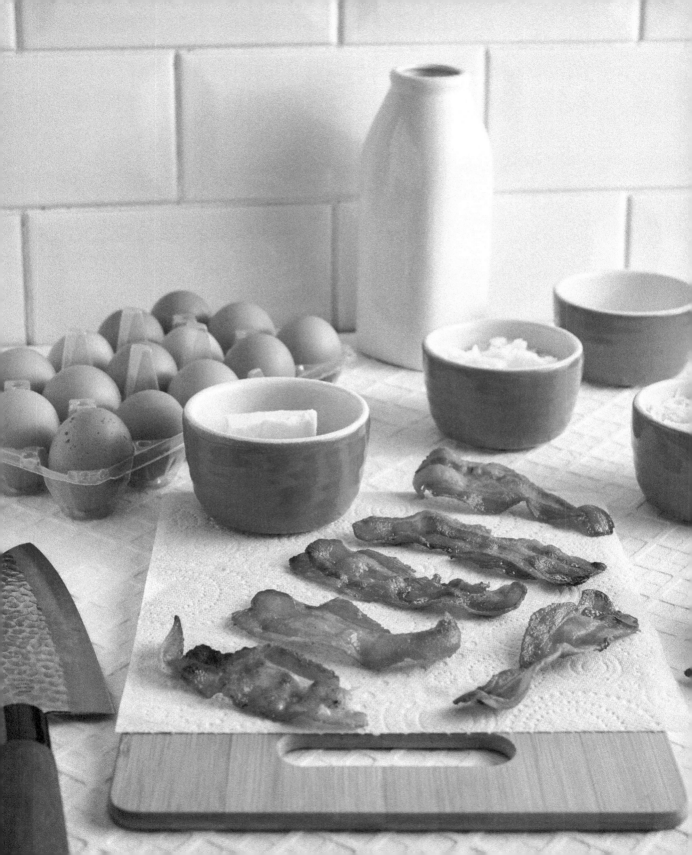

# HIGH FAT, LOW CARB, SUPER EASY

Whether you are a keto newbie or a veteran, if you haven't discovered the combination of keto and meal prep, then your life is about to be changed once again. The great thing about keto is the ability to adapt your diet and lifestyle to any situation. You can always find something packaged or on a menu that is keto-friendly. But that also can limit your progression if you are constantly eating out or eating highly processed foods. Taking things back to the kitchen and preparing healthy and nutritious home-cooked meals will take you and your goals to the next level.

# My Keto Philosophy

When I started researching what a ketogenic diet was, it seemed intimidating, hard to comprehend, and limited. As I studied, lived it, and felt the benefits, I realized how wrong I was. Keto became maintainable once I felt comfortable in the aisles of the grocery store and cooking in the kitchen. I know you'll be able to relate, too, as you gain confidence limiting carbohydrates and incorporating healthy fats into your diet. I hope the material within these pages will provide the most cost-friendly, easy-to-prepare, enjoyable meal prep possible. For me, easy meal prep is the only way I can be consistent with my family, budget, and time.

With keto, reaching your macros is key. In this book the daily macros we are looking to reach are 5 to 10 percent carbs, 15 to 30 percent protein, and 60 to 75 percent fat. By following these recipes and meal prep plans, you can easily hit these goals and implement the keto lifestyle into your own with ease.

I was nervous about my first book, *The One-Pot Ketogenic Diet Cookbook*, being too basic and the recipes too simple. When I received so much positive feedback about that being the main reason readers loved it most, I was elated! In this day and age you can read anything on the Internet and get conflicting information at every turn. My goal with this book (and my philosophy in general) is to simplify this transformative lifestyle so it is doable, stress-free, and easy to maintain and adapt for years to come.

# Keto Staple Foods

When I first committed to keto, I spent a ton of time figuring out what I could and couldn't eat and what I should and shouldn't buy. I knew that keto was ideally based on consuming whole, unprocessed, single-ingredient foods. I read labels, researched, and made discoveries by trial and error. I still believe that buying organic products is best, but I know that's not always practical in the monthly food budget. Buy the best quality of meats, eggs, dairy products, and vegetables your pocketbook allows.

Enjoy a variety of meat, fish, eggs, full-fat dairy products like cheeses, butter, and cream, low-carb nuts (especially pecans, macadamia nuts, brazil nuts, walnuts, almonds, and pine nuts), healthy oils, low-carb condiments, low-carb veggies like broccoli, cauliflower, and leafy greens—and a whole lot of avocados! Here's a more detailed list of these ketogenic kitchen staples, which you will see are called for frequently in this book's recipes.

**Avocados.** Avocados are a ketogenic diet staple. They are low in carbs, packed full of nutrients, and high in healthy fats. They pair well with most dishes and are a great way to add flavor and fat into your diet.

**Dairy.** Full-fat dairy products, including cream cheese, sour cream, cheeses, heavy (whipping) cream, and grass-fed butter make any dish creamy and rich, and they are all keto approved. Avoid dairy products with added sugars as well as those that are low-fat and fat-free. Even though dairy is a key aspect of the ketogenic lifestyle, you can still manage to do a dairy-free keto diet. Some tips that accompany the recipes in this book can help you pull this off.

**Eggs.** Eggs are convenient, inexpensive, and easy to add to any dish. You can fry, scramble, poach, and boil eggs. Having a dozen eggs in the refrigerator at all times is a great way to stay on track and always have a backup meal plan. Half an avocado, bacon, and a couple of fried eggs is the perfect keto meal. Use free-range and organic eggs when possible.

**Fats and oils.** Olive oil, avocado oil, coconut oil, MCT oil, lard, beef tallow, butter, and ghee are healthy fats that should be incorporated into your diet. Cooking meats and vegetables in these healthy fats helps you achieve your keto goals by making your meals filling and satisfying. When you are keto-adapted, these healthy fats are your body's primary fuel source, so it's important to add these fats to your diet.

**Meats.** When it comes to meats, you can eat pretty much whatever you want—just be sure to balance lean meats with fatty side dishes to hit your macros with every meal. Watch for added sugars in bacon and sausages and stick to uncured and no-sugar-added meats.

**Nut Flours**. Almond and coconut flour are great keto substitutes for wheat flour. Both are gluten-free, grain-free, and low-carb. When making keto-friendly desserts, baked goods, or breading for proteins, these flours are great to have on hand.

**Nuts**. Nuts and nut butters in moderation are a great fat source. Stick to nuts that are high in fat and low in carbs like almonds, macadamia nuts, walnuts, and pecans. Watch out for pistachios, cashews, and sunflower seeds due to their higher carb content. Nuts are very calorie-dense, so watch your serving size.

**Salt**. When living a ketogenic lifestyle, you may experience a decrease in sodium. Adding extra salt to your food may be scary at first, but it is essential when going low carb. Ideally, use Himalayan salt or sea salt.

**Sweeteners**. Stevia and erythritol are all-natural, low-carb sugar replacements. Experiment to see what tastes best to you and what your body responds well to. When you are craving something sweet or need to take your Fat Coffee (page 78) to the next level, it's nice to have these on hand so you can keep your blood sugar stable and your sweet tooth satisfied.

**Vegetables**. When shopping in the produce section, stick to mostly green vegetables. Choose non-starchy veggies like broccoli, cabbage, cauliflower, lettuce, zucchini, and Brussels sprouts. Stay away from starchy vegetables like beans, corn, potatoes, and winter squashes.

## FOODS TO LIMIT

You may enjoy certain higher-carb fruits and vegetables in moderation. For instance, a handful of berries or a small serving of squash, carrots, tomatoes, or onions are okay to incorporate into your diet. I cook with a few of these ingredients often, because I love the flavor and texture they bring to my dishes. I feel it's worth using some of my daily carbs to enjoy their contribution.

Watch for higher carbs in cottage cheese, full-fat yogurts with added sugar, and certain nuts, including cashews, chestnuts, and pistachios, and their corresponding nut flours. These items are fine to incorporate into your diet in moderation, just be sure to track those carbs.

# KETO FLU

By default, our bodies burn carbohydrates or glucose as energy. When you transition into a ketogenic lifestyle and drastically decrease your carb intake, your body is depleted of stored glucose. This metabolic process is called ketosis, which is when our body uses fatty acid or ketones as energy. This can be a bit of a shock for our bodies, and many people respond with flu-like symptoms, which we typically refer to as the keto flu. The keto flu will hit some much harder than others.

Common symptoms of the keto flu are:

- Nausea
- Irritability
- Brain fog
- Stomach pains

- Heart palpitations
- Muscle cramping
- Sugar cravings
- Trouble focusing

Please don't let these symptoms scare you. Can you imagine what your body is going through as it transitions from using glucose as energy to using fat instead? Stay with it for at least four to six weeks and be patient. The first two to three weeks should be the worst of it. Trust the process and you'll never look back.

Symptoms of the keto flu are likely to pop up when you are dehydrated or experience electrolyte loss and withdrawal from carbs or sugar. You can greatly reduce your risk and reaction to symptoms by doing these things:

- Drink plenty of water
- Replenish lost electrolytes; supplement with potassium, magnesium, and sodium
- Sip on bone broth
- Increase your salt intake
- Exercise

- Try your best to get at least eight hours of sleep
- Take exogenous ketone supplements—I believe in taking these if you're just beginning your ketogenic journey

After taking care of your physical needs, give yourself time to adjust adjust. You're going through a big transition. Try to be patient and kind with yourself, and don't stress too much about calories. Focus on keeping your carbs low and your fat high, which is exactly what this book is designed to help you do.

Foods to altogether avoid on a keto diet include grains, most fruits, processed foods, starchy vegetables, sugary drinks, and refined fats.

Watch nutrition labels for hidden sugars and carbs while grocery shopping and cooking. This is especially important when you are buying condiments, sauces, and dressings rather than making them yourself. Store-bought versions of these products are often loaded with sweeteners and starchy thickeners.

Alcohol should also be avoided, but dry wines and low-carb spirits can be consumed in small amounts. When you drink alcohol, your body is going to burn the alcohol first as energy and then use fat (if you are fat adapted). So, realize when you are drinking that you aren't making any progress, just stalling until your body burns through the alcohol.

# The Benefits of Meal Prep

There are many reasons that lead people to meal prep. These are the top reasons I do it:

**Saves time**. Instead of prepping dinner from scratch on weeknights and scrambling to find something for lunch when you're late for work, you can be prepared when you make the time for meal prepping over the weekend. Spend your weeknights with your family and friends and not messing up and cleaning the kitchen over and over again.

**Saves money**. Meal prep means no more expensive meals out (save those for the weekend) when you are in a crunch. By making the time and planning ahead for meal prep, you won't be tempted to make a quick and unhealthy decision to swing by the drive-through. With the shopping lists in the meal prep chapters you'll buy just what you need, which saves you money.

**Portion control**. Having prepped meals that are portioned out will prevent you from overeating. It helps me maintain my drive to stay on track living keto.

**Weeknight success.** In *The One-Pot Ketogenic Diet Cookbook*, I provided one-pot meals that can be made within 30 minutes to keep nights as stress-free as possible. With this book, I am taking it one step further by eliminating weeknight prep. Making the time on the weekend to have a stress-free week is worth dirtying the kitchen just once a week.

**Multitasking skills.** I will help you on this one with the step-by-step plans I've provided in each of the six different meal preps. This will give you the skills to find your own routine and execute kitchen prep work in the most effective and efficient way possible.

# Meal Prep Principles

The most important part of all of this is *planning ahead* and blocking out time for cooking, which is much easier said than done. Trust me, I get it. However, making the effort to plan ahead will save you time and energy, and it will pay off in the long run with results you can see and feel.

Most importantly, meal prep is going to help you reach your goals and discover your best self by helping you follow a healthy and consistent routine and avoid the temptation of unhealthy quick and easy choices. Having already-prepped meals in your refrigerator for a quick grab-and-go will do wonders for your nutrition and goals. It is very difficult to diet successfully and maintain healthy lifestyle changes because most nutritious foods require some type of preparation. We are hardwired to take the easiest route and choose what is quickest and most convenient.

### START SIMPLE

The most important part of meal prep is keeping it simple and stress-free. There is no need to prep extravagant meals with unfamiliar ingredients. In part 3's Staples section (page 77), I have given you the foundation ingredients and how to prep them. My hope is that when you get through my preps you will have the tools to create your own simple preps in the future to keep you on track with your goals.

### INGREDIENT REUSE

I am a sucker for sales and saving as much money as I can at the checkout. When my family was in the middle of a move and didn't have a kitchen for a time, we ate out for almost every meal. I did the best I could at keeping my meals keto-compliant. When I realized how much we were spending on fast food, though, I was just sick. The amount of money you can save when you plan ahead, reuse ingredients in multiple meals, and keep it basic will shock you. This way of life isn't just good for your body and mind but your bank account as well.

### BATCH COOK

If you are new to keto, don't let the stress of a single meal prep intimidate you. I promise this way of life will save you so much potential stress throughout the week. My biggest piece of advice is to sit down and plan ahead before you actually start cooking. Hopefully the step-by-steps I have provided in the preps will help you with this. And be patient with your multitasking skills in the kitchen. The more you cook multiple things at once, the better you will get at it.

### FIND YOUR RHYTHM

My personal execution consists of sitting down with a pen and paper and planning the meals I'd like to prep. I keep in mind what will stay fresh and good throughout the week, as well as what is on sale in my local grocery store. Then I order my shopping list according to my route around the store. Once I have completed my shopping trip, I sit down again with a pen and paper and figure out my plan of attack for my weekend prep. I think about how I can reuse bowls or pans where possible, if I can bake anything at the same time, and the steps I will take to make the most of my time in the kitchen. I make sure I have enough time to let the food cool before I seal up the containers and store them in the refrigerator.

# INTERMITTENT FASTING

Intermittent fasting is a pattern of eating where you alternate between a period of fasting and a period of eating. How you incorporate this into your nutrition plan depends on your goal. Intermittent fasting benefits include:

- Improved mental clarity
- Increased energy
- Improved insulin sensitivity
- Increased blood ketones
- Fat loss

Intermittent fasting can be implemented in a number of ways. A couple of the most common include:

**16:8** You will eat all your meals within an 8-hour time period and fast the remaining 16 hours. This can be done daily or a few days a week. This is my favorite fasting protocol because research has found that restricting eating to 8 or 9 hours does not negatively impact your ability to maintain or build muscle. My husband practices 16:8 intermittent fasting 4 to 5 days a week, and he is in the best shape he's been in in years. He's put on lean muscle mass, and his immune system has improved tremendously, as well as his mental health. He even works out while fasting! Our workouts used to be controlled by food and timing, but our lives have now become so much less stressful.

**20:4** You will eat all your meals within a 4-hour eating window and fast the remaining 20 hours. This protocol will likely prevent muscle gain while increasing fat loss.

While fasting, you want to be sure to stay hydrated. Approved liquids to drink while fasting include:

- Exogenous ketones (ketones taken as supplements)
- Water
- Black coffee
- Tea
- Bone broth

# The Art of Storage

I hope that meal prep will become a regular routine in your home like it is in ours. In order to make that happen, it is essential that you invest in and choose the right storage containers. When I was ready to invest in a set of containers, I bought a few different options—glass, metal, and plastic (BPA-free, of course). This way I could do a trial run to figure out what I liked best before I made a big purchase. Trying a few to see what you like and what works best in your kitchen will save you time and money in the long run.

## CONTAINERS

Good-quality containers are essential for keeping your food fresh as long as possible. Here are some things to look for when buying containers for meal prepping:

**BPA-free.** I'm sure you have read or seen BPA-free on containers or other plastic items before, and here's why it's important. BPA stands for bisphenol A, which is a chemical found in plastics like food containers, water bottles, food cans, and consumer goods. Research has shown that BPA can seep into food or beverages from plastic containers made of BPA. Possible side effects of BPA exposure include increased blood pressure, mental health issues, and negative effects on fetuses, infants, and children.

**Stackable.** I know we all have a cupboard or a drawer packed full of containers and lids. If you begin to make meal prep a part of your regular routine, that means a lot of containers will start to accumulate. Having containers that are stackable will keep your cupboards functional and looking organized, making life easier.

**Freezer-safe.** There will be times when you prep and have more than you need for the week. That's when having containers that are freezer-safe is key. I will also purposely double recipes so I can throw them in the freezer for future use.

**Microwave-safe.** It is totally up to you how you reheat your meals. Most likely microwaving is going to be the most convenient method. So, choosing containers that are microwave-friendly is something you will want to pay attention to.

**Dishwasher-safe.** This one is obvious, at least it is for me.

## GLASS CONTAINERS

In our house we use glass containers for many reasons. Glass is environmentally friendly. It performs safely at different temperatures, allowing me to reheat meals in the prep containers right in the microwave or oven. Although glass is a little more of an investment than plastic, with glass containers you get safety and durability. They also don't retain any of the smells of food after cleaning, which is a nice bonus. Square, rectangular, and circular glass containers are available; choose a mixture of sizes for the most versatility.

## PLASTIC CONTAINERS

Plastic containers are very popular for meal prep—they're lightweight, stack easily, and many are now microwavable as well as freezable. But as I mentioned, my go-to is glass. Plastic containers may leach harmful substances into the food stored in them. Plastic is not biodegradable, which means it isn't possible for our earth to naturally absorb the material back into the soil; instead, plastic actually contaminates it. Unlike glass and metal, plastic absorbs odors and tastes like whatever you stored in it previously. If you have ever stored fish in a plastic container, I'm guessing it still smells like fish to this day. While it's a fact that plastic is cheaper than other options, it's also true that it will not last as long. If you do choose to go with plastic containers, always look for an indicator that they are BPA-free.

## MASON JARS

Mason (canning) jars are also great for storing food. Made of glass, Mason jars are inexpensive and perfect for storing salads and salad dressings. A combination of wide-mouth quart and pint jars, as well as some smaller four-ounce jars for dressings, will go a long way when doing meal preps. I incorporate them a few times throughout the preps for quick storage.

## STAINLESS STEEL

Stainless steel containers will last a lot longer than plastic. They look nicer, maintain hot and cold temperatures well, and are super durable. They are the most expensive option, and one drawback to keep in mind is that metal can't be reheated in the microwave.

Whichever type of storage container you decide to purchase, I recommend getting at least 15 containers as well as five pint-size or quart-size Mason jars so you have enough storage for your meals through one week of prep.

## SMART LABELING

I didn't worry about labeling foods with the date purchased or prepared until I realized how much food I was throwing out. The problem was that I thought I would remember when I bought everything and use it before it went bad. When I started labeling and meal prepping, I became a lot more aware of what was in the refrigerator and when I needed to use it by, which meant saving money.

I always keep a roll of freezer tape and a permanent marker in a drawer in the kitchen. I like to put the "best by" date so I know exactly how long each meal is good for.

## THAWING

The best way to defrost frozen food is to place the frozen item in the refrigerator to thaw. This does require thinking ahead and giving yourself enough time to have it thawed before you are ready to enjoy it.

The cold-water thawing method can be quicker than defrosting in the refrigerator but requires more attention. The food must be in a leakproof bag and submerged in cold water. Replace the water every 30 minutes until thawed.

It's not recommended to freeze and reheat fish. It will last up to four days in the refrigerator.

## REHEATING

Microwaving is the most convenient and quickest way to reheat food. I always reheat meals in one-minute intervals until I reach my desired temperature, sometimes at 60 percent power. Keep a close eye on your meal and stir it occasionally for an even temperature throughout.

You can also reheat your meals using the oven or a grill. Another option would be heating a skillet on the stovetop over medium heat and emptying the prepped meal into the skillet, stirring until you've reached the desired temperature.

When reheating leftovers, look for an internal temperature of 165°F.

# FOOD STORAGE CHART

| FRESH MEATS | FRIDGE | FREEZER |
|---|---|---|
| Salads, eggs, fish | 1 TO 2 DAYS | DOES NOT FREEZE WELL |
| Beef, pork, lamb | 1 TO 2 DAYS | 3 TO 4 MONTHS |
| Bacon | 7 DAYS | 1 MONTH |
| Poultry | 1 TO 2 DAYS | 9 TO 12 MONTHS |

| COOKED MEATS | FRIDGE | FREEZER |
|---|---|---|
| Salads, eggs, fish | 3 TO 5 DAYS | DOES NOT FREEZE WELL |
| Beef, pork, lamb | 3 TO 5 DAYS | 3 TO 6 MONTHS (UP TO 12 MONTHS FOR ROASTS) |
| Bacon | 7 DAYS | 1 MONTH |
| Poultry | 3 TO 5 DAYS | 2 TO 4 MONTHS |

When buying meats and dairy from your local grocery store, look for products with the "sell by" date farthest in the future. It may take some digging, but the food products will store longer for your meal prep.

Make sure to let your prepped meals completely cool before you cover them and put them in the refrigerator or freezer. If you don't wait and put the lid on while the meal is still hot, it will create steam within your storage container. This will result in the meal continuing to cook, which can lead to overcooked vegetables or dried-out proteins.

# Kitchen Equipment

I am all about keeping the kitchen stocked with only the essential items. Below are what I consider the must-haves and the nice-to-haves.

MUST-HAVE

The list below might look long, but I'm betting you have nearly everything already. I'm including everything on this list not only to make sure you have it but also to illustrate why each of these items is so helpful for meal prepping.

**Chef's knife.** If you have only used a cheap knife in the past, changing to a quality chef's knife will be a game changer.

**Skillet.** Try to choose one that can go from stovetop to oven (cast iron preferred). Being able to use one piece of equipment for multiple tasks is only going to save you time. I use a cast-iron skillet almost daily because I can brown meat in it on the stovetop, sauté veggies, and then pour eggs over the top and put it in the oven.

**Sheet pan.** Having a few sheet pans is smart for meal prep so you can have multiple preps going at once. I mainly use rimmed 13-by-18-inch aluminum sheet pans.

**Measuring cups and measuring spoons**. These are essential for measuring ingredients.

**Colander**. Great for rinsing fruit and vegetables and draining boiled broccoli or green beans.

**Cutting board**. You have several different options when it comes to a good cutting board. I personally use a wood block instead of a plastic cutting board because wood doesn't score as deeply as plastic does and lasts longer if cared for properly. To care for wood cutting boards, start with a clean and thoroughly dry cutting board. Apply mineral oil with a paper towel or cloth and let dry for a few hours, or overnight if possible.

**Saucepans**. Having a few sizes of saucepans is useful, especially when preparing multiple meals at once.

**Spiralizer**. This is key when living a low-carb lifestyle. You'll use it to make veggie noodles. There are many options available in a wide range of prices starting at less than $10. Amazon is your friend.

**Muffin tin**. A muffin tin (standard size, 12 cup) is great for making dishes in premeasured single servings. For example, we will use one in the first week of the beginner's prep for Ham and Cheese Breakfast Muffins (page 26).

**Mason jars**. We use a lot of mason jars at our house. We use them for drinking glasses, to make dressings, and to store meal-prep salads. I have sets of 12-, 16-, and 24-ounce jars that we use regularly. I also have a few four-ounce jars that I use to store homemade salad dressings.

**Food storage containers**. As we talked about earlier, there are several options when it comes to meal-prep containers. In each prep we have three or four different meals for five days total. I would recommend getting at least 20 containers to store your meal preps for each week.

**Countertop or immersion blender**. Having one of these is crucial for an amazing cup of frothy Fat Coffee (page 78), for blending dressings, and for puréeing soups or vegetables.

**Digital thermometer.** A digital thermometer is a must-have in the kitchen and will change the quality of your meals. So much can vary in cook methods and recipes, so being able to monitor the internal temperature of whatever you are cooking is crucial. Making an instant-read thermometer part of your cooking and baking routine will allow you to control the tenderness and texture of everything you put on the table.

**Baking dish.** Having a few baking dishes in the kitchen and doing meal prep go hand in hand. Using them to prep everything from large breakfast casseroles to one-pot meals will keep the dirty dishes to a minimum. I like to use glass baking dishes so I can watch the contents cook, and so I can cook, serve, refrigerate, and freeze all in the same dish.

### NICE-TO-HAVE

What you see included here makes my life easier. Are these items necessary? No. Do they help me eat keto well throughout the year? Absolutely.

**Traeger Wood Pellet Grill.** This may be an odd piece of equipment to add to the list but let me tell you why I included it. I developed the recipes in this book in the dead of summer with no air-conditioning, and my pellet grill prevented me from heating the house up. Anything you cook or bake in your kitchen you can do on this grill.

**Food scale.** I would really like to add this to the must-haves list, but you don't need this until you start creating your own preps. I am a huge advocate of tracking calories and macronutrients, and using a digital food scale is a must when you want to take it to the next level.

# This Book's Meal Preps

I wanted to offer options for all types of people following the ketogenic diet, so I created three different meal preps to support your different needs and goals. Each prep will provide two weeks of preps with three or four recipes in each week. So, altogether, you will have eight weeks of structured meal prep and meal plans that will focus on simple, doable, and flavorful recipes. In part 3, I have meal prep-friendly breakfast, lunch, and dinner recipes to help you create your own meal preps as you continue living this lifestyle.

**Beginner's Prep**—This prep is directed toward people who are in the beginning stages of keto. No matter what your goals are, this prep will assist in getting you into ketosis, keeping you there, and promoting fat loss and mental clarity. There is no fasting in this prep, and it will include breakfast recipes.

**Performance Prep**—This prep is for those who live an active lifestyle and want to support that way of life by living keto. I incorporated intermittent fasting or fat coffee, a dairy-free prep, and a little more protein due to your fat-adapted status.

**Maintenance Prep**—Have you met your performance and fat loss goals? Then this prep is for you. Sometimes once we reach our goals it's easy to fall back into our old ways quickly. Please recognize how great you feel in ketosis and commit to the lifestyle.

If you are sensitive to dairy, know that there are often easy substitutions for dairy products in my recipes. I've given you tips for dairy-free cooking throughout the book.

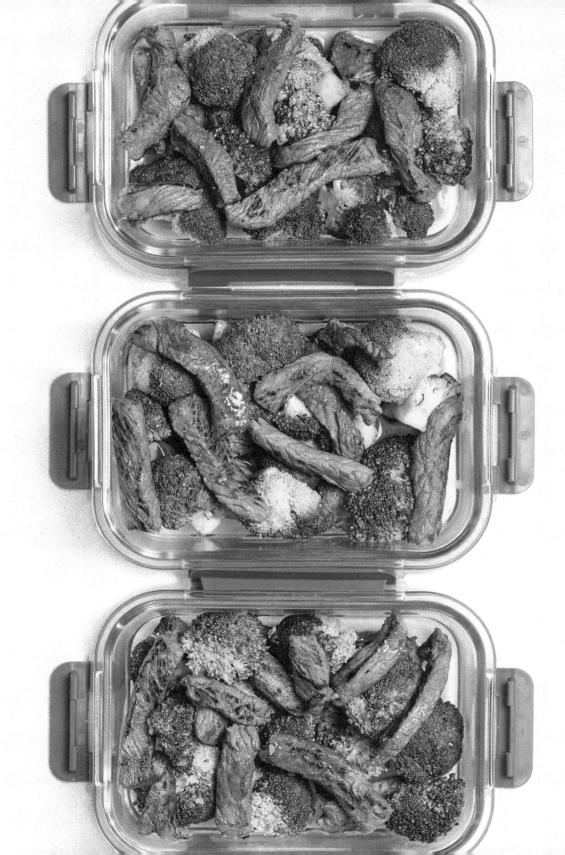

# PART TWO

# KETO MEAL PREP PLANS & RECIPES

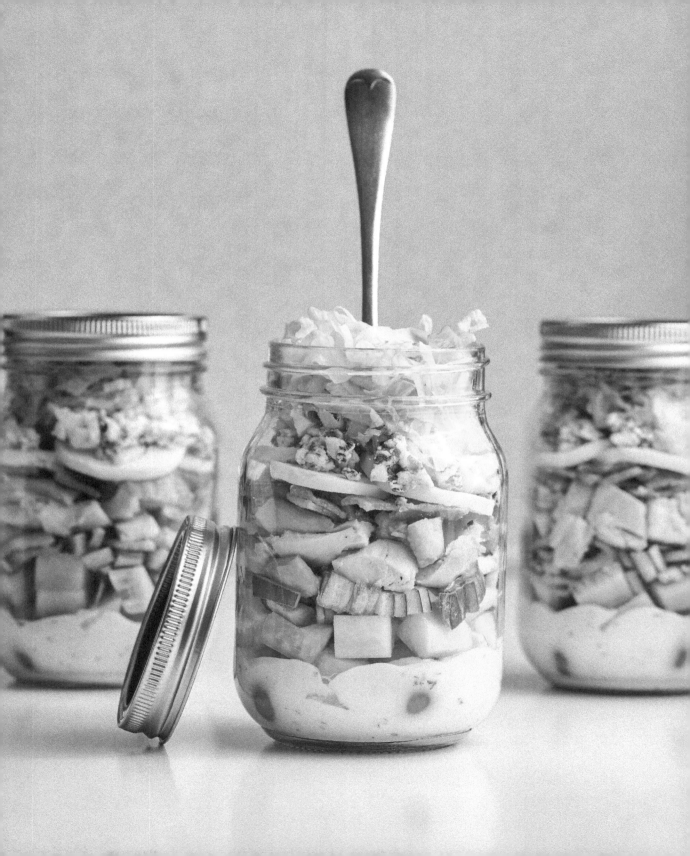

# BEGINNER'S MEAL PREP

Meal prep and beginning to follow a keto lifestyle go hand in hand. My goal is to provide you with the tools for a successful, low-stress start on the ketogenic diet. The first week of meal prep includes a breakfast recipe to satisfy you in the morning. In the second week I call for Fat Coffee (page 78) for your first "meal" of the day. Fat Coffee is incredibly satiating, but it's not something you can prep in advance. It's very simple and quick to make in the morning, as long as you have the needed ingredients on hand. The meals may seem a little bit repetitive when you are just starting out, but saving the extra time you would have spent cooking and entering your meals into a macro counter is well worth it.

I did my best to keep the shopping lists simple and easy on the wallet. If you don't already have some of the pantry staples, the first few shopping trips may cost a little more than usual. Remember, all fats are not created equal, so splurge on healthy fats such as coconut oil, grass-fed butter, and avocado oil.

## Week 1

Ham and Cheese Breakfast Muffins **26**

Cobb Salad **28**

Chicken Egg Salad Wraps **30**

Blue Cheese Bacon Burgers **31**

## Week 2

Fajita Salad **34**

Chicken Parmesan over Zucchini Noodles **36**

Italian Zucchini Boats **38**

Fat Coffee **78**

<< Cobb Salad (page 28)

# BEGINNER'S WEEK 1

## SHOPPING LIST

### PANTRY

- Apple cider vinegar
- Avocado oil
- Black pepper, ground
- Coconut milk, full-fat (1 [13.6-ounce] can)
- Dijon mustard
- Garlic powder
- Mayonnaise (1 [24-ounce] jar)
- Nonstick cooking spray
- Onion powder
- Salt
- Worcestershire sauce

### PRODUCE

- Broccoli (8 ounces)
- Celery stalks (3)
- Cucumbers (2)
- Garlic (2 cloves)
- Grape tomatoes (1 pint)
- Lemon (1)
- Lettuce, butter leaf (1 head)
- Lettuce, romaine (2 heads)
- Parsley (1 bunch)
- Red onion (1)
- Tomato (1)

### PROTEIN

- Beef, ground (1½ pounds)
- Chicken thighs, boneless and skinless (1¼ pounds)
- Uncured bacon (8 ounces)
- Ham, cooked (6 ounces)
- Eggs, large (2 dozen)

### DAIRY

- Cheddar cheese (4 ounces)
- Blue cheese crumbles (4 ounces)

## EQUIPMENT

- Baking sheets (2)
- Chef's knife
- Cutting board
- Measuring cups and spoons
- Mixing bowl
- Muffin tin
- Storage containers (16)
- Whisk

## STEP-BY-STEP PREP

1. Follow step 1 of the Blue Cheese Bacon Burgers (page 31) and refrigerate the patties. Wash the bowl well to use in preparation for the breakfast muffins.

2. Preheat the oven to 400°F.

3. Follow steps 1 and 2 of the Hard-boiled Eggs recipe (page 82).

4. Prepare the ingredients for the Ham and Cheese Breakfast Muffins (page 26) and follow steps 1 through 5.

5. Follow steps 1 and 2 of the Perfectly Cooked Bacon (page 79) and steps 1 and 2 of the Baked Boneless Chicken Thighs (page 80).

6. Prepare the Dairy-Free Ranch Dressing (page 90) and refrigerate.

| | BREAKFAST | LUNCH | DINNER |
|---|---|---|---|
| **DAY 1** | Ham and Cheese Breakfast Muffins | Blue Cheese Bacon Burgers | Cobb Salad |
| **DAY 2** | Ham and Cheese Breakfast Muffins | Chicken Egg Salad Wraps | Blue Cheese Bacon Burgers |
| **DAY 3** | Ham and Cheese Breakfast Muffins | Cobb Salad | Chicken Egg Salad Wraps |
| **DAY 4** | Ham and Cheese Breakfast Muffins | Cobb Salad | Chicken Egg Salad Wraps |
| **DAY 5** | Ham and Cheese Breakfast Muffins | Blue Cheese Bacon Burgers | Cobb Salad |

7. Check on the breakfast muffins and hard-boiled eggs. Remove the muffins when done and follow recipe steps 5 and 6.

8. Reduce the oven temperature to 375°F. Place the prepared sheets of bacon and chicken thighs in the oven to bake.

9. Prepare the romaine, cucumbers, onions, and celery for the Cobb Salad (page 28) and Chicken Egg Salad Wraps (page 30) and set aside.

10. Check on the bacon and chicken. When done, transfer the bacon to a paper towel-lined plate to drain. Remove the chicken from the oven to cool when cooked through.

11. Prepare the Cobb Salad (page 28) steps 1 through 3.

12. Finish the Blue Cheese Bacon Burgers (page 31) steps 2 and 3.

13. Prepare the Chicken Egg Salad Wraps (page 30).

# HAM AND CHEESE BREAKFAST MUFFINS

**MAKES 5 SERVINGS**

PREP TIME: 10 minutes    COOK TIME: 15 minutes

This recipe for breakfast muffins is such a great option for meal prep and an on-the-go lifestyle. It is easy to throw together, requires minimal cleanup, and the muffins are great hot or cold. This recipe also allows you to get creative with other ingredient combinations such as spinach, mushrooms, and mozzarella, or bacon, Cheddar, and bell peppers.

Nonstick cooking spray

15 large eggs

Salt

Freshly ground black pepper

½ teaspoon onion powder

½ teaspoon garlic powder

1½ cups chopped broccoli

1 cup cubed ham

1 cup shredded Cheddar cheese

½ cup diced tomatoes

1 teaspoon Dijon mustard

1. Preheat the oven to 400°F. Spray 15 cups of 2 muffin tins with cooking spray or line with silicone liners.

2. In a large mixing bowl, crack the eggs and season them with salt, pepper, onion powder, and garlic powder. Using a whisk, mix well.

3. Add the broccoli, ham, cheese, tomatoes, and mustard to the bowl and mix well.

4. Divide the egg mixture evenly into the prepared muffin cups, filling each about two-thirds full.

5. Bake for 15 minutes, until set. Let cool.

6. Into each of 5 storage containers, place 3 muffins.

**Storage:** Place the airtight containers in the refrigerator for up to 5 days or freeze for 3 months. To thaw, refrigerate overnight. Serve cold or reheat in the microwave for 1 to 2 minutes.

> **MAKE IT DAIRY-FREE:** Skip the cheese and add ¼ cup of full-fat coconut cream in its place.

> **SERVING TIP:** Serve with salsa, avocado, and/or sour cream if desired.

Per Serving: Calories: 364; Total Fat: 23g; Protein: 30g; Total Carbs: 10g; Net Carbs: 7g; Fiber: 3g; Sodium: 956mg

**Macros: 57% Fat; 33% Protein; 10% Carbs**

# COBB SALAD

**MAKES 4 SERVINGS**

PREP TIME: 20 minutes

COOK TIME: 0 minutes (with precooked bacon, chicken, and eggs on hand) or 30 minutes (if cooking bacon, chicken, and eggs)

A hearty Cobb salad is a low-carb dieter's dream and the perfect salad to order at a restaurant or to incorporate in your meal prep. If you aren't a blue cheese fan, feta is always a great alternative.

2 romaine lettuce heads, chopped

2 cups chopped Baked Boneless Chicken Thighs (page 80)

1 cup grape tomatoes

2 cucumbers, diced

½ cup chopped red onion

4 slices Perfectly Cooked Bacon (page 79), chopped

½ cup crumbled blue cheese

4 Hard-boiled Eggs (page 82), sliced

½ cup Dairy-Free Ranch Dressing (page 90)

**1.** Evenly divide the lettuce between 4 storage containers.

**2.** Evenly distribute and arrange the chicken, tomatoes, cucumbers, onion, bacon, blue cheese, and eggs over the lettuce.

**3.** Divide the dressing into 2-tablespoon servings and store on the side.

**Storage:** Place the airtight containers in the refrigerator for up to 5 days.

**STORAGE TIP:** You can also store your salads in a mason jar to cut out the extra container for the dressing. The first layer on the bottom will be the dressing, then the tomatoes, cucumbers, onion, chicken, bacon, eggs, blue cheese, and lettuce. Put the lid on and refrigerate. When ready to serve, shake the jar and enjoy.

**MAKE IT DAIRY-FREE:** Omit the blue cheese.

Per Serving: Calories: 545; Total Fat: 38g; Protein: 33g; Total Carbs: 23g; Net Carbs: 20g; Fiber: 3g; Sodium: 1,098mg

**Macros: 63% Fat; 24% Protein; 13% Carbs**

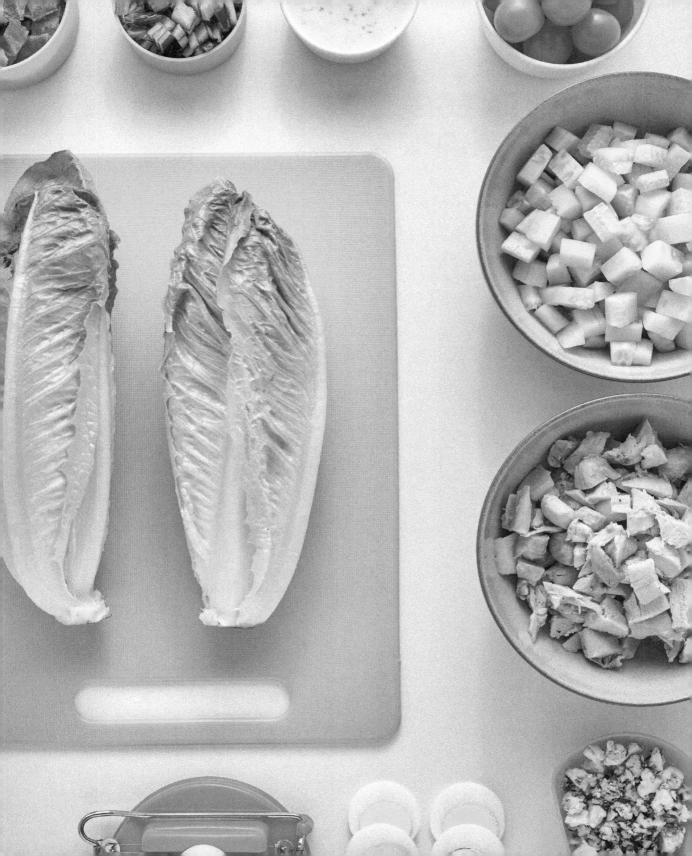

# CHICKEN EGG SALAD WRAPS

**MAKES 3 SERVINGS**

PREP TIME: 10 minutes

COOK TIME: 0 minutes (with precooked chicken and eggs on hand) or 30 minutes (if cooking chicken and eggs)

In this recipe, I tried to keep the prep as simple and budget-friendly as possible. If you have the chicken thighs and eggs already prepped, you can have this whipped up in no time. You will also be using the chicken and hard-boiled eggs in the Cobb Salad (page 28) prep. If you don't have those items prepped, the cook time will be around 30 minutes.

1½ cups chopped Baked Boneless Chicken Thighs (page 80)

6 Hard-boiled Eggs (page 82), chopped

3 celery stalks, minced

2 tablespoons minced red onion

1 tablespoon Dijon mustard

2 cups Mayonnaise (page 87)

Salt

Freshly ground black pepper

8 leaves butter or romaine lettuce

1.　In a large bowl, combine the chicken, eggs, celery, onion, and mustard. Add the Mayonnaise and stir until mixed. Season with salt and pepper.

2.　Divide the egg salad and lettuce between 3 storage containers. To serve, make egg salad wraps by filling the lettuce leaves with the salad and wrapping the lettuce around it.

**Storage:** Place the airtight containers in the refrigerator for up to 4 days.

**VARIATION TIP:** For extra flavor, add a bit of curry powder to your egg salad.

**MAKE IT VEGETARIAN:** Skip the chicken and add 2 additional eggs to make this recipe vegetarian.

Per Serving: Calories: 1,202; Total Fat: 122g; Protein: 22g; Total Carbs: 3g; Net Carbs: 2g; Fiber: 1g; Sodium: 1,398mg

**Macros: 91% Fat; 7% Protein; 2% Carbs**

# BLUE CHEESE BACON BURGERS

**MAKES 4 SERVINGS**

PREP TIME: 10 minutes, plus refrigeration time    COOK TIME: 12 minutes

One of my favorite ways to enjoy a burger is with bacon and blue cheese. This recipe is simplified by incorporating the cheese and bacon right into the patty, rather than layering them on top separately. If you aren't a blue cheese fan, don't shy away from this recipe. Just add a slice of your favorite cheese to the top of the burgers when they are almost done cooking.

1½ pounds ground beef

4 slices Perfectly Cooked Bacon (page 79), crumbled

½ cup crumbled blue cheese

1 tablespoon Worcestershire sauce

2 large eggs

Salt

Freshly ground black pepper

1 romaine lettuce head, chopped

1 avocado, chopped

1 cup grape tomatoes

**1.** In a large mixing bowl, combine the beef, bacon, blue cheese, Worcestershire sauce, and eggs. Season with salt and pepper. Use your hands to shape 4 patties. Cover with plastic and refrigerate for 30 minutes to 2 hours.

**2.** Heat the grill or broiler on high and cook for 4 to 5 minutes on each side, or until the burgers are cooked to your liking. Remove from the grill and let cool.

**3.** Into each of 4 storage containers, divide the lettuce, avocado, and tomatoes, and top with a burger patty.

**Storage:** Place the airtight containers in the refrigerator for up to 5 days. The patties can be served hot or cold. Reheat the burgers separately from the other ingredients for 1 to 2 minutes in the microwave or in a 400°F oven for 8 to 10 minutes.

**VARIATION TIP:** Avocado-Lime Dressing (page 91) would be a good addition to this recipe.

Per Serving: Calories: 772; Total Fat: 54g; Protein: 61g; Total Carbs: 10g; Net Carbs: 6g; Fiber: 4g; Sodium: 1,107mg

**Macros: 63% Fat; 31% Protein; 6% Carbs**

# BEGINNER'S WEEK 2

## SHOPPING LIST

### PANTRY

- Black pepper, ground
- Chicken broth (1 [14.5-ounce] can)
- Coconut oil
- Cumin
- Erythritol
- Extra-virgin olive oil
- Garlic powder
- Marinara sauce, low carb (1 [16-ounce] jar)
- Onion powder
- Oregano, dried
- Paprika
- Pork rinds (2 cups)
- Red pepper flakes
- Salt
- Vanilla extract

### FRESH PRODUCE

- Avocado (1)
- Bell pepper, green (1)
- Bell pepper, red (1)
- Chicken broth (1 [14.5-ounce] can)
- Cilantro, fresh (1 bunch)
- Lettuce, romaine (1 head)
- Limes (3)
- Onions, yellow (2)
- Zucchini (6)

### PROTEIN

- Chicken thighs, bone-in (3)
- Flank steak (1 [2-pound] steak)
- Italian sausage, bulk (1 pound)
- Eggs, large (2)

### DAIRY

- Salted butter (1 stick)
- Cheddar cheese (½ cup or 2 ounces)
- Heavy (whipping) cream (1 pint)
- Parmesan cheese, grated (1 cup or 4 ounces)
- Sour cream (1 [8-ounce] container)

## EQUIPMENT

- Baking dish
- Rimmed baking sheet
- Chef's knife
- Cutting board
- French press/coffee maker
- Ice cube tray or silicone molds
- Immersion blender
- Measuring cups and spoons
- Mixing bowls
- Skillet
- Storage containers (11)
- Vegetable spiralizer

## STEP-BY-STEP PREP

1. Marinate the flank steak in step 1 of the Fajita Salad (page 34).

2. Preheat the oven to 375°F.

3. Follow steps 1 through 4 for the Chicken Parmesan (page 36) and prep the Zucchini Noodles (page 83).

4. Prep the Italian Zucchini Boats (page 38) through step 5.

5. Using the same skillet you used to prep the mixture for the boats, prepare the onions and peppers for the Fajita Salad (page 34) in step 3.

| | BREAKFAST | LUNCH | DINNER |
|---|---|---|---|
| **DAY 1** | Fat Coffee | Chicken Parmesan over Zucchini Noodles | Fajita Salad |
| **DAY 2** | Fat Coffee | Fajita Salad | Italian Zucchini Boats |
| **DAY 3** | Fat Coffee | Italian Zucchini Boats | Chicken Parmesan over Zucchini Noodles |
| **DAY 4** | Fat Coffee | Fajita Salad | Italian Zucchini Boats |
| **DAY 5** | Fat Coffee | Chicken Parmesan over Zucchini Noodles | Fajita Salad |

**6.** Check on the chicken and when done, remove and let cool. Reduce the oven temperature to 350°F and bake the zucchini boats following step 6.

**7.** Check on the zucchini boats and when done, let cool before packing into storage containers.

**8.** Turn the broiler to high and follow step 2 of the Fajita Salad (page 34).

**9.** Follow steps 5 and 6 of the Chicken Parmesan over Zucchini Noodles (page 36).

# FAJITA SALAD

**MAKES 4 SERVINGS**

PREP TIME: 20 minutes, plus marinating time    COOK TIME: 10 minutes

I can't stress enough how worth it it is to make your marinade and let the flank steak marinate in it overnight. If you're doing your meal prep on Sunday, for instance, make the marinade on Saturday night to give the steak plenty of marinating time. Thin slices of the steak will really add flavor to your meals throughout the week. It's also great with eggs served with sautéed vegetables (in fat, of course) for dinner.

**FOR THE STEAK**

1 (2-pound) flank steak

¼ cup extra-virgin olive oil

1 teaspoon garlic powder

1 teaspoon onion powder

1 teaspoon ground cumin

Juice of 1 lime

1 bunch cilantro,
   leaves chopped

Salt

Freshly ground black pepper

**FOR THE SALAD**

2 tablespoons extra-virgin
   olive oil or coconut oil

1 yellow onion, sliced

1 green bell pepper, sliced

1 red bell pepper, sliced

6 cups chopped
   romaine lettuce

½ cup sour cream

½ cup shredded
   Cheddar cheese

2 limes, quartered

1 avocado

**TO MAKE THE STEAK**

1.  In a large resealable bag, add the flank steak, oil, garlic powder, onion powder, cumin, lime juice, cilantro, salt, and pepper. Marinate for 30 minutes to 24 hours.

2.  When ready to cook, turn the broiler on high and remove the flank steak from the marinade, discarding the remaining marinade. Place the steak on a baking sheet and bake for 3 to 5 minutes on each side. Let rest for 10 minutes before thinly slicing against the grain.

**TO MAKE THE SALAD**

1.  Heat a large skillet over medium heat and combine the oil, onion, and peppers. Stir often and cook until the onion becomes translucent, 8 to 10 minutes.

2.  Into each of 4 divided storage containers, place the steak, peppers, and onions in one side, and the lettuce, sour cream, cheese, and lime wedges in the other side. Before enjoying an individual serving, halve, pit, and chop an avocado. Top the steak with ¼ of the chopped avocado, along with the lettuce, sour cream, and cheese. Squeeze the lime juice over everything and mix.

**Storage:** Place the airtight containers in the refrigerator for up to 5 days. If desired, reheat the peppers and beef in a separate container in the microwave for 1 to 2 minutes.

**SUBSTITUTION TIP:** To switch this recipe up, you could use chicken or shrimp instead of steak, or do a combination of both.

**MAKE IT DAIRY-FREE:** Skip the sour cream and cheese and don't skimp on the avocado.

Per Serving: Calories: 893; Total Fat: 60g; Protein: 70g; Total Carbs: 17g; Net Carbs: 11g; Fiber: 6g; Sodium: 480mg

**Macros: 60% Fat; 31% Protein; 9% Carbs**

# CHICKEN PARMESAN OVER ZUCCHINI NOODLES

**MAKES 3 SERVINGS**

PREP TIME: 10 minutes   COOK TIME: 40 minutes

Zucchini noodles are going to be your best friend on keto. Pre-keto, my favorite food was chicken Parmesan with pasta, and now I can enjoy it minus the heavy starches. The best part about the dish is the hearty chicken. Now I substitute zucchini noodles for the pasta and I still get to enjoy this amazing rich sauce and stay within my goals.

**FOR THE CHICKEN**

2 cups crushed pork rinds

¼ cup grated
   Parmesan cheese

Salt

Freshly ground black pepper

2 large eggs

3 bone-in chicken thighs

1 teaspoon garlic powder

3 tablespoons extra-virgin
   olive oil

**FOR THE NOODLES**

3 cups Zucchini Noodles
   (page 83)

1½ cups low-carb
   marinara sauce

Salt

Freshly ground black pepper

1.   Preheat the oven to 375°F.

2.   In a shallow dish, stir together the pork rinds and Parmesan cheese. Season with salt and pepper. In a separate dish, whisk the eggs.

3.   Pat the chicken dry using a paper towel and dip each piece in the egg, then in the pork rind mixture. Repeat.

4.   In a large ovenproof skillet (preferably cast iron), heat the oil over medium heat. Add the chicken thighs and cook on each side for 6 to 7 minutes. Let them cook fully on each side before flipping or moving them.

5.   Arrange the chicken in the skillet and bake for 25 to 30 minutes, until the internal temperature reaches 165°F.

6.   Into each of 3 storage containers, pack 1 cup zucchini noodles, ½ cup marinara, and 1 chicken thigh.

**Storage:** Place the airtight containers in the refrigerator for up to 5 days. To reheat, microwave for 1 to 2 minutes or bake in a 400°F oven for 8 to 10 minutes.

**INGREDIENT TIP:** When searching for a low-carb marinara sauce, start with the label and check the carb content, fiber, and the ingredient list. Whichever has the least amount of ingredients and carbs is the way to go.

**MAKE IT DAIRY-FREE:** Simply omit the Parmesan cheese.

Per Serving: Calories: 649; Total Fat: 42g; Protein: 45g; Total Carbs: 25g; Net Carbs: 19g; Fiber: 6g; Sodium: 1,565mg

**Macros: 58% Fat; 28% Protein; 14% Carbs**

# ITALIAN ZUCCHINI BOATS | MAKES 3 SERVINGS

PREP TIME: 10 minutes     COOK TIME: 40 minutes

Don't be afraid to get creative with these preps, especially if Italian isn't your thing. You could pair Baked Boneless Chicken Thighs (page 80) and broccoli, turn it into a taco-style boat with ground beef and Mexican seasonings, or fill the zucchini with Bolognese (page 45).

3 zucchini, halved lengthwise

1 tablespoon avocado oil

1 medium onion, diced

2 tablespoons minced garlic

1 pound ground
    Italian sausage

2 teaspoons paprika

1 teaspoon red pepper flakes

2 teaspoons dried oregano

1 cup chicken broth

¾ cup grated
    Parmesan cheese

Salt

Freshly ground black pepper

1.   Preheat the oven to 350°F.

2.   Using a spoon, scoop out the flesh of each zucchini half and chop it up.

3.   In a large skillet, heat the oil over medium heat. Sauté the onion, garlic, and sausage, cooking until browned, 6 to 8 minutes. Add the chopped zucchini flesh, paprika, red pepper flakes, and oregano.

4.   Fill the prepped zucchini shells with equal portions of the sausage mixture. Place them in a 9-by-13-inch baking dish and pour the broth into the bottom of the dish.

5.   Top with the Parmesan cheese and season with salt and pepper. Cook for 30 to 35 minutes, until the cheese is bubbling.

6.   Into each of 3 storage containers, place 2 zucchini halves.

**Storage:** Place the airtight containers in the refrigerator for up to 5 days. Reheat in the microwave for 1 to 2 minutes or in a 400°F oven for 8 to 10 minutes.

Per Serving: Calories: 720; Total Fat: 55g; Protein: 44g; Total Carbs: 15g; Net Carbs: 11g; Fiber: 4g; Sodium: 2,061mg

**Macros: 69% Fat; 24% Protein; 7% Carbs**

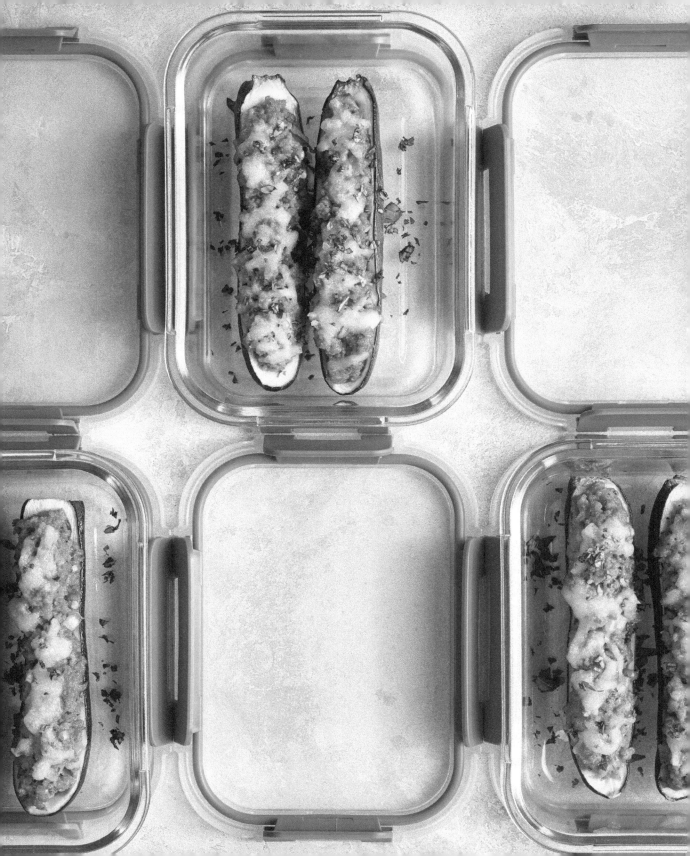

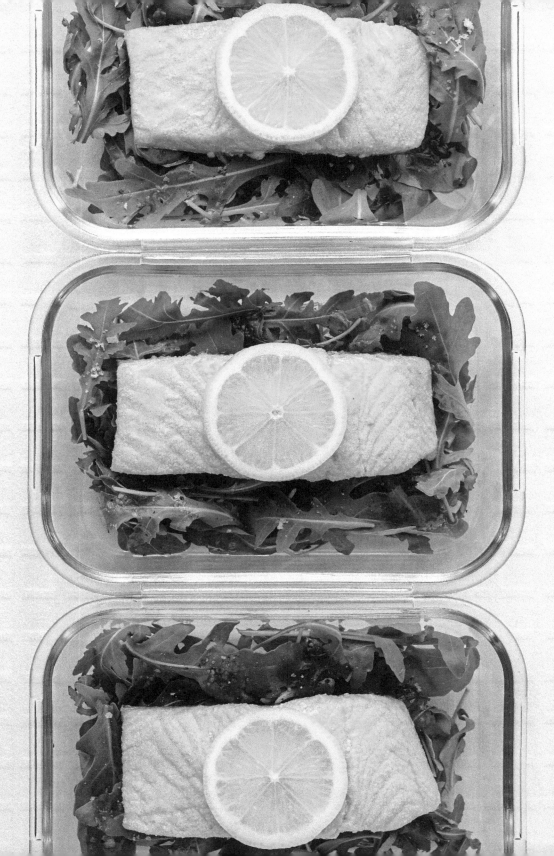

# PERFORMANCE MEAL PREP

I've created this performance meal prep plan to set you up for nutritional success. My husband and I run a gym together in Wyoming, and we often hear from people who think time in the gym can make up for a bad diet. That is just not the case. I am the most passionate about this prep because, if I stick to it, I don't end up sacrificing my gym time. It helps me keep my diet and my workout regimen consistent. The goal with this performance meal prep is to eliminate body fat while maintaining lean body mass. I have eliminated dairy and increased the protein for these two weeks. It is common for dairy to cause inflammation. By cutting it from your diet, you may see an increase in your rate of fat loss. Pay attention to how your body feels in response to taking out dairy and consuming more protein instead. Don't be afraid to train while fasting. Skip that post-workout protein shake and throw out your scale; body circumference measurements are much more telling.

## Week 1

Ground Beef and Cabbage Stir-Fry **44**

Bolognese over Spaghetti Squash **45**

Arugula and Salmon Salad **46**

Fat Coffee **78**

## Week 2

Mason Jar Breakfast Pudding **50**

Beef and Broccoli Stir-Fry **51**

Bratwursts and Sauerkraut **54**

Roasted Chicken over Pesto Spaghetti Squash **55**

« Arugula and Salmon Salad (page 46)

# PERFORMANCE WEEK I

## SHOPPING LIST

### PANTRY

- Apple cider vinegar
- Black pepper, ground
- Coconut aminos
- Coconut oil
- Erythritol
- Extra-virgin olive oil
- Garlic powder
- Garlic salt
- Oregano, dried
- Salt
- Tomato paste (1 [6-ounce] can)
- Tomatoes, diced, low sugar (1 [14.5-ounce] can)

### PRODUCE

- Arugula (8 ounces)
- Bell pepper, green (1)
- Cabbage, green (1 head)
- Celery stalks (2)
- Garlic (2 cloves)
- Lemon (1)
- Onion, yellow (1)
- Scallions (4)
- Squash, spaghetti (1 [4-pound])

### PROTEIN

- Beef, ground (2½ pounds)
- Salmon (3 [4-ounce] fillets)

## EQUIPMENT

- Baking dish
- Baking sheet
- Chef's knife
- Cutting board
- Measuring spoons and cups
- Skillet
- Storage containers (11)

## STEP-BY-STEP PREP

1.  Prep the fresh vegetables for the Ground Beef and Cabbage Stir-Fry (page 44) and the Bolognese over Spaghetti Squash (page 45).

2.  Preheat the oven to 450°F and follow steps 1 through 3 of the Arugula and Salmon Salad (page 46).

3.  When the salmon is done cooking, remove it from the oven, and reduce the oven temperature to 350°F. Finish assembling the salmon salad.

| | BREAKFAST | LUNCH | DINNER |
|---|---|---|---|
| **DAY 1** | Intermittent fasting or Fat Coffee | Bolognese over Spaghetti Squash | Ground Beef and Cabbage Stir-Fry |
| **DAY 2** | Intermittent fasting or Fat Coffee | Ground Beef and Cabbage Stir-Fry | Arugula and Salmon Salad |
| **DAY 3** | Intermittent fasting or Fat Coffee | Arugula and Salmon Salad | Bolognese over Spaghetti Squash |
| **DAY 4** | Intermittent fasting or Fat Coffee | Bolognese over Spaghetti Squash | Ground Beef and Cabbage Stir-Fry |
| **DAY 5** | Intermittent fasting or Fat Coffee | Ground Beef and Cabbage Stir-Fry | Arugula and Salmon Salad |

**4.** Cut the spaghetti squash lengthwise and remove the seeds. Place the halves, cut-side down, in a baking dish and fill the bottom with ¼ inch of water. Bake for 45 to 50 minutes, or until tender. Remove from the oven and let cool. Use a fork to remove the spaghetti-like strands from the squash.

**5.** Follow steps 1 through 4 of the Bolognese over Spaghetti Squash (page 45).

**6.** Heat a large skillet over medium heat and follow steps 1 through 4 of the Ground Beef and Cabbage Stir-Fry (page 44).

# GROUND BEEF AND CABBAGE STIR-FRY

**MAKES 4 SERVINGS**

PREP TIME: 15 minutes    COOK TIME: 20 minutes

I never appreciated cabbage until I started the ketogenic diet. Now it's one of my go-to low-carb vegetables! I love shredded cabbage for salads, and there is nothing tastier than sautéed cabbage with butter and salt. Cabbage is a nutrient-dense blank canvas and super filling. The coconut aminos (aka keto soy sauce) and apple cider vinegar add great flavor to this dish.

1 tablespoon coconut oil

1½ pounds ground beef

2 garlic cloves, minced

1 green cabbage head, cored and chopped

2 tablespoons coconut aminos

2 tablespoons apple cider vinegar

Salt

Freshly ground black pepper

4 scallions, both white and green parts, chopped

Sesame seeds (optional)

Sriracha (optional)

Toasted sesame oil (optional)

**1.** In a large skillet, heat the oil over medium heat. Cook the beef and garlic until the beef is browned, 5 to 7 minutes.

**2.** Add the cabbage to the skillet and continue to cook until the cabbage becomes slightly wilted, 8 to 10 minutes.

**3.** Add the coconut aminos and vinegar and season with salt and pepper.

**4.** Evenly divide the stir-fry between 4 storage containers. To serve, top with the scallions, and with the sesame seeds, sriracha, and toasted sesame oil, if using.

**Storage:** Place the airtight containers in the refrigerator for up to 5 days. Reheat in the microwave for 1 to 2 minutes or in a 400°F oven for 8 to 10 minutes.

**SUBSTITUTION TIP:** You could swap out the ground beef and use pork sausage instead, or use a mix of the two.

Per Serving: Calories: 550; Total Fat: 33g; Protein: 49g; Total Carbs: 13g; Net Carbs: 8g; Fiber: 5g; Sodium: 641mg

**Macros: 54% Fat; 36% Protein; 10% Carbs**

# BOLOGNESE OVER SPAGHETTI SQUASH

**MAKES 4 SERVINGS**

PREP TIME: 10 minutes    COOK TIME: 45 minutes

You will notice in my recipes that I use garlic powder or garlic salt frequently. If time isn't an issue, of course minced fresh garlic always is better. Dishes like this one would be even better if you sautéed fresh garlic with the butter and onions, but with busy schedules, the extra step of incorporating fresh garlic isn't always realistic.

1 tablespoon extra-virgin olive oil

1 yellow onion, chopped

2 celery stalks, finely chopped

1 green bell pepper, chopped

1 pound ground beef

2 tablespoons tomato paste

1 (14.5-ounce) can diced tomatoes, drained

1 tablespoon erythritol

1 tablespoon dried oregano

1 teaspoon garlic powder

Salt

Freshly ground black pepper

1 recipe Spaghetti Squash (page 86)

**1.**   In a large skillet over medium heat, heat the oil. Add the onion, celery, and bell pepper and sauté, stirring frequently, 6 to 8 minutes, or until softened. Once the veggies are cooked down, add the ground beef and brown until cooked through, about 10 minutes more.

**2.**   Stir in the tomato paste, tomatoes, erythritol, oregano, garlic powder, salt, and pepper. Bring to a boil and simmer on low for 20 to 30 minutes, stirring occasionally.

**3.**   Let the sauce cool.

**4.**   Divide the spaghetti squash between 4 storage containers and top each with Bolognese sauce.

**Storage:** Place the airtight containers in the refrigerator for up to 7 days. Reheat for 1 to 2 minutes in the microwave or in a 375°F oven for 8 to 10 minutes.

> **COOKING TIP:** The longer you let the sauce simmer, the better the flavors will develop. That makes it great as a meal prep option, as it gets even better as the days go by.

Per Serving: Calories: 415; Total Fat: 24g; Protein: 33g; Total Carbs: 21g; Net Carbs: 18g; Fiber: 3g; Sodium: 372mg

**Macros: 52% Fat; 32% Protein; 16% Carbs**

# ARUGULA AND SALMON SALAD

**MAKES 3 SERVINGS**

PREP TIME: 15 minutes    COOK TIME: 10 minutes

When living a ketogenic lifestyle, your diet is often heavy in omega-6 fatty acids, which are found in nuts, oils, chicken thighs, and eggs. It's important to balance those with omega-3 fatty acids because it's a little more difficult to get omega-3 fatty acid from your diet on keto. Salmon is a great source of omega-3 fatty acid and should be a staple in your ketogenic lifestyle.

3 (4-ounce) salmon fillets

5 tablespoons extra-virgin olive oil, divided

1 teaspoon garlic salt

Juice of 1 lemon

4½ cups arugula

1. Preheat the oven to 450°F. Line a baking sheet with aluminum foil.

2. Rub the fillets with 2 tablespoons of oil and the garlic salt. Place them on the prepared sheet and drizzle the lemon juice over the top of the fillets.

3. Bake until the salmon is cooked through and flaky, 8 to 12 minutes. Let the fillets rest for 10 minutes.

4. Into each of 3 storage containers, place 1½ cups of arugula and season with salt and pepper. Top the arugula with the salmon fillets. To serve, drizzle the arugula in each container with 1 tablespoon of oil and toss.

**Storage:** Place the airtight containers in the refrigerator for 4 days. Serve cold or, to reheat, remove the salmon and reheat it in the microwave for 1 to 2 minutes or in a 400°F oven for 5 to 6 minutes.

> **INGREDIENT TIP:** A key thing I've learned about cooking salmon is to avoid overthinking it. A little olive oil, freshly squeezed lemon juice, salt, and pepper go a long way. If the skin is on, you'll cook them skin-side down. Salmon cooks quickly, so don't stray too far from the oven, and start checking the fillets for doneness after about 8 minutes.

Per Serving: Calories: 393; Total Fat: 31g; Protein: 26g; Total Carbs: 6g; Net Carbs: 4g; Fiber: 2g; Sodium: 91mg

**Macros: 71% Fat; 26% Protein; 3% Carbs**

# PERFORMANCE WEEK 2

## SHOPPING LIST

### PANTRY

- Almonds, sliced
- Avocado oil
- Black pepper, ground
- Chia seeds
- Chicken broth (1 [14.5-ounce] can)
- Cinnamon, ground
- Coconut aminos
- Coconut cream or full-fat unsweetened coconut milk (1 [5-ounce] can)
- Coconut, unsweetened, shredded
- Flaxseed
- Garlic powder
- Hemp hearts
- Onion powder
- Pesto sauce (¼ cup)
- Salt
- Sauerkraut (1 [16-ounce] jar)
- Sesame oil
- Stevia
- Vanilla extract

### PRODUCE

- Broccoli (2 crowns)
- Garlic (3 cloves)
- Ginger (1-inch piece)
- Onion, yellow (1)
- Spaghetti squash (1 [4-pound])

### PROTEIN

- Sirloin steak (1½ pounds)
- Bratwurst sausage (1 pound)
- Chicken thighs, bone-in (4)

## EQUIPMENT

- Baking sheet
- Chef's knife
- Colander
- Cooking pot
- Cutting board
- Measuring cups and spoons
- Mixing bowls
- Saucepan
- Skillet
- Storage containers (17)

## STEP-BY-STEP PREP

1.  Follow the directions to marinate the beef for the Beef and Broccoli Stir-Fry (page 51).

2.  Preheat the oven to 375°F and follow steps 2 through 5 of the Roasted Chicken over Pesto Spaghetti Squash (page 55).

3.  While the chicken is baking, in a medium saucepan, follow steps 1 and 2 of the Mason Jar Breakfast Pudding (page 50).

4.  Check on the chicken. When done, let it cool, and reduce the oven to 350°F. Prepare the Spaghetti Squash (page 86).

| | BREAKFAST | LUNCH | DINNER |
|---|---|---|---|
| **DAY 1** | Mason Jar Breakfast Pudding | Bratwursts and Sauerkraut | Beef and Broccoli Stir-Fry |
| **DAY 2** | Mason Jar Breakfast Pudding | Beef and Broccoli Stir-Fry | Roasted Chicken over Pesto Spaghetti Squash |
| **DAY 3** | Mason Jar Breakfast Pudding | Roasted Chicken over Pesto Spaghetti Squash | Beef and Broccoli Stir-Fry |
| **DAY 4** | Mason Jar Breakfast Pudding | Bratwursts and Sauerkraut | Roasted Chicken over Pesto Spaghetti Squash |
| **DAY 5** | Mason Jar Breakfast Pudding | Beef and Broccoli Stir-Fry | Bratwursts and Sauerkraut |

5. Prepare the Bratwursts and Sauerkraut (page 54).

6. Bring a large pot of water to a boil, heat a large skillet, and follow steps 1 through 5 of the Beef and Broccoli Stir-Fry (page 51).

7. Check on the squash and complete steps 6 and 7 of the Roasted Chicken over Pesto Spaghetti Squash (page 55).

# MASON JAR BREAKFAST PUDDING

**MAKES 5 SERVINGS**

PREP TIME: 10 minutes    COOK TIME: 20 minutes

In the performance prep, we are cutting out dairy, and for some people that can be difficult because so many of their fats are dairy sourced. My favorite way to swap out cream is with canned coconut cream or coconut milk. To whip the coconut cream, refrigerate the can overnight, which will allow the coconut cream to rise to the top and solidify. Scoop out the cream, avoiding the watery liquid in the bottom, and whip until it's fluffy and forms peaks.

2 (13.6-ounce) cans unsweetened coconut milk or coconut cream

¼ cup unsweetened shredded coconut

¼ cup hemp hearts

3 tablespoons chia seeds

3 tablespoons flaxseed

3 teaspoons stevia

Pinch salt

Pinch ground cinnamon

2 teaspoons vanilla extract

¼ cup sliced almonds

**1.**    In a medium saucepan, mix the coconut milk, coconut, hemp hearts, chia seeds, flaxseed, stevia, salt, and cinnamon. Bring to a boil. Reduce the heat and let simmer on low, whisking continuously, until thickened, about 8 to 10 minutes.

**2.**    Remove from the heat and add the vanilla.

**3.**    Divide the mixture evenly between 5 mason jars. Top each jar with sliced almonds.

**Storage**: Place the airtight jars in the refrigerator for up to 6 days.

**STORAGE TIP:** Taking advantage of mason jars with meal prep is very budget friendly. You can purchase a 12-pack of 16-ounce mason jars for less than $20.

Per Serving: Calories: 397; Total Fat: 39g; Protein: 7g; Total Carbs: 8g; Net Carbs: 5g; Fiber: 3g; Sodium: 52mg

**Macros: 88% Fat; 7% Protein; 5% Carbs**

# BEEF AND BROCCOLI STIR-FRY

**MAKES 4 SERVINGS**

PREP TIME: 15 minutes, plus marinating time    COOK TIME: 10 minutes

Blanching broccoli is the best way to make sure it still has a little bite to it. This cooking method will keep the vegetable bright green and help maintain its crisp texture—which is especially important for meal prep. My favorite way to finish off blanched broccoli is in a hot skillet with butter, garlic, and salt.

**FOR THE MARINADE**

6 tablespoons coconut aminos

¼ cup avocado oil

2 tablespoons toasted sesame oil

1 teaspoon garlic powder

1 teaspoon onion powder

Salt

Freshly ground black pepper

1½ pounds sirloin steak, cut into ¼-inch-thick slices

**FOR THE BEEF AND BROCCOLI**

1 teaspoon salt, plus more for seasoning

2 broccoli crowns, florets separated and trimmed

2 tablespoons avocado oil

3 garlic cloves, minced

1 tablespoon finely minced ginger or ½ tablespoon ground ginger

¼ cup coconut aminos

¼ cup toasted sesame oil

Freshly ground black pepper

**TO MAKE THE MARINADE**

In a bowl, combine the coconut aminos, avocado oil, sesame oil, garlic powder, onion powder, salt, and pepper. Add the steak and toss to coat. Marinate for at least 30 minutes or up to 24 hours in the refrigerator.

**TO MAKE THE BEEF AND BROCCOLI**

1.   Fill a large pot halfway with water and add 1 teaspoon of salt. Bring to a boil.

2.   Add the broccoli and blanch for 1 to 3 minutes; drain in a colander. Rinse with cold water to prevent further cooking. Set aside.

3.   Heat a large skillet over medium-high heat and combine the avocado oil, garlic, and ginger and cook for 30 seconds.

4.   Add the sliced beef, discarding the marinade, and cook, stirring constantly, for 2 to 3 minutes. Add the broccoli, coconut aminos, and sesame oil to the skillet and season with salt and pepper. Continue to cook until the beef has reached your desired doneness (about 5 to 7 minutes for medium).

5.   Divide the stir-fry evenly between 4 storage containers.

CONTINUED

**Storage:** Place the airtight containers in the refrigerator for up to 5 days or freeze for 3 months. To thaw, refrigerate overnight. Reheat for 1 to 2 minutes in the microwave or in a 375°F oven for 8 to 10 minutes.

**COOKING TIP:** I used to associate marinating meat with extra work and thought it was overrated. I have developed an appreciation for this simple step that adds a ton of flavor to the final product. It's all about thinking ahead and letting the meat sit with a few simple ingredients overnight. The flavor of the finished dish is well worth the extra step; you'll be able to taste the difference.

Per Serving: Calories: 588; Total Fat: 38g; Protein: 54g; Total Carbs: 6g; Net Carbs: 4g; Fiber: 2g; Sodium: 1,177mg

**Macros: 58% Fat; 37% Protein; 5% Carbs**

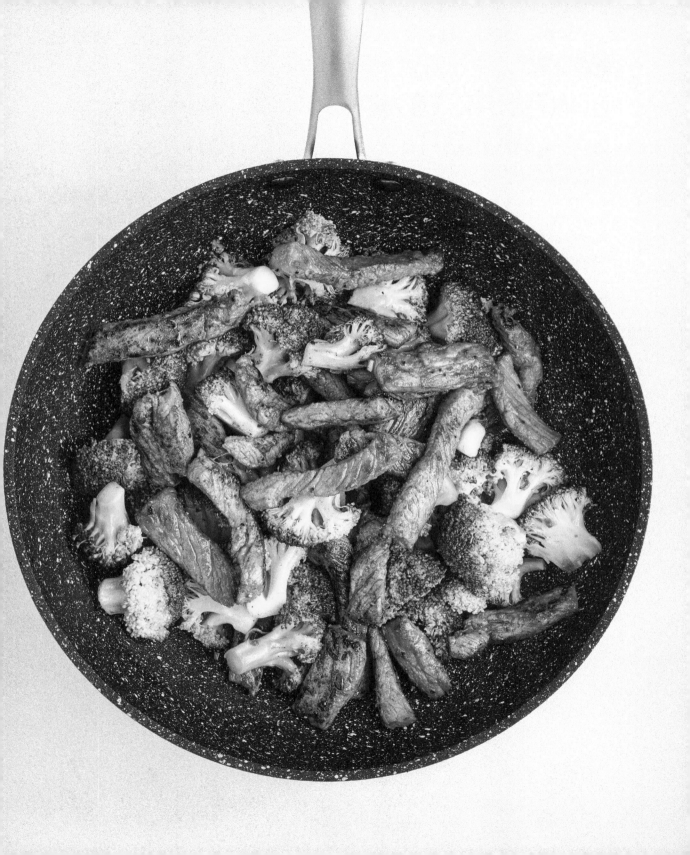

# BRATWURSTS AND SAUERKRAUT

**MAKES 4 SERVINGS**

PREP TIME: 10 minutes    COOK TIME: 40 minutes

I like to incorporate fermented foods into my diet to promote gut health and keep my carb intake low. If you're not making your own fermented foods, buy a jar at your local grocery store for naturally fermented sauerkraut.

2 tablespoons avocado oil

1 yellow onion, thinly sliced

1 pound bratwurst

1 (16-ounce) jar sauerkraut, drained

1½ cups chicken broth

1 teaspoon garlic powder

Salt

Freshly ground black pepper

1. In large cast-iron skillet over medium heat, add the oil, onion, and bratwurst and cook for 6 to 8 minutes, or until they get some color.

2. Add the sauerkraut, broth, garlic powder, salt, and pepper and simmer for 30 to 40 minutes, or until the sausages are cooked through.

3. In each of 4 storage containers, place 1 cup of sauerkraut and 1 bratwurst.

**Storage:** Place the airtight containers in the refrigerator for up to 5 days or freeze for 3 months. To thaw, refrigerate overnight. Reheat in the microwave for 1 to 2 minutes or in a 375°F oven for 8 to 10 minutes.

Per Serving: Calories: 525; Total Fat: 42g; Protein: 24g; Total Carbs: 12g; Net Carbs: 8g; Fiber: 4g; Sodium: 2,994mg

**Macros: 72% Fat; 18% Protein; 10% Carbs**

# ROASTED CHICKEN OVER PESTO SPAGHETTI SQUASH

**MAKES 4 SERVINGS**

PREP TIME: 15 minutes    COOK TIME: 30 minutes

This may be one of my favorite meals for preps, as you can't go wrong with the pesto spaghetti squash. Make sure to not overcook it when reheating, to keep it a little firm.

4 (3- to 4-ounce) bone-in chicken thighs

¼ cup extra-virgin olive oil

1 teaspoon garlic powder

1 teaspoon onion powder

Salt

Freshly ground black pepper

1 recipe Spaghetti Squash (page 86)

¼ cup prepared pesto sauce (see Ingredient Tip)

1. Preheat the oven to 375°F.

2. Pat the chicken thighs dry with paper towels and place them in a shallow dish.

3. Add the oil, garlic powder, and onion powder. Season with salt and pepper. Mix until the chicken is coated evenly.

4. Place the seasoned chicken on a baking sheet, making sure the skin is wrapped around the thigh.

5. Bake for 30 to 40 minutes, or until the chicken has reached an internal temperature of 165°F.

6. In a medium bowl, toss together the spaghetti squash and pesto sauce. Season with salt and pepper, and combine until the squash is evenly coated.

7. Divide the squash noodles between 4 storage containers and top each with a chicken thigh. Let cool and secure the lids.

**Storage:** Place the airtight containers in the refrigerator for up to 6 days or freeze for 3 months. To thaw, refrigerate overnight. Reheat in the microwave for 1 to 2 minutes or in a 375°F oven for 8 to 10 minutes.

**INGREDIENT TIP:** Making your own pesto is pretty dang easy if you have the right ingredients on hand and a food processor. All you need is fresh basil, garlic, pine nuts, salt, pepper, and olive oil.

Per Serving: Calories: 361; Total Fat: 30g; Protein: 18g; Total Carbs: 6g; Net Carbs: 6g; Fiber: <1g; Sodium: 447mg

**Macros: 75% Fat; 20% Protein; 5% Carbs**

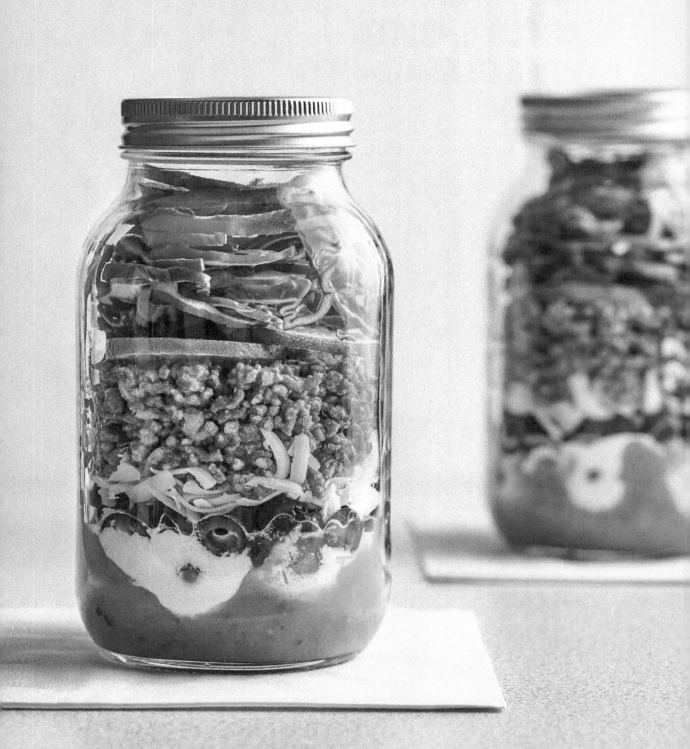

# MAINTENANCE MEAL PREP

Once you have reached your goal weight, keeping it off can sometimes be harder than losing it was. Remember that the ketogenic diet is a lifestyle, not a quick fix. In this maintenance prep we add a little bit more protein and calories while continuing to keep carbs as low as possible. The most important piece is the low-carb aspect, so don't stress as much about meeting your fat and protein goals. Now that you are fat-adapted, feel free to experiment and see how flexible your body is within ketosis. If you decide to play around with carb counts, choose whole, unprocessed carbohydrates (such as sweet potatoes). The best time to eat carbs is post-workout or after physical activity. Continue to steer clear of refined and processed carbs. Listen closely to your body to discover what it responds to best, and then give it that.

## Week 1

Chicken Caesar Salad **60**

Taco Salad **61**

Chicken Drumsticks and Cauliflower Rice **62**

Fat Coffee **78**

## Week 2

Breakfast Frittata **67**

Sheet Pan Meat Loaf with Green Beans **69**

Glazed Balsamic Salmon Salad **71**

Low-Carb Chili **73**

◀◀ Taco Salad (page 61)

# MAINTENANCE WEEK 1

## SHOPPING LIST

### PANTRY

- Anchovy paste
- Beef broth (1 [14.5-ounce] can)
- Black olives, sliced (1 [16-ounce] can)
- Extra-virgin olive oil
- Garlic salt
- Onion powder
- Salsa, low carb/sugar (1 cup)
- Taco seasoning
- Worcestershire sauce
- Yellow mustard, prepared

### FRESH PRODUCE

- Cabbage, green (1 head)
- Cauliflower (1 head)
- Garlic (2 cloves)
- Grape tomatoes (1 pint)
- Lemon (1)
- Lettuce, romaine (1 head)
- Limes (2)
- Onion, red (1)
- Onion, yellow (1)

### PROTEIN

- Beef, ground (1 pound)
- Chicken drumsticks (6)
- Chicken thighs, boneless, skinless (12 ounces)
- Eggs, large (6)

### DAIRY

- Cheddar cheese, shredded (1 ¼ cups or 5 ounces)
- Heavy (whipping) cream (1 pint)
- Parmesan cheese, grated (½ cup or 2 ounces)
- Salted butter (½ cup or 1 stick)
- Sour cream (1 [8-ounce] container)

## EQUIPMENT

- Chef's knife
- Cutting board
- Mason jars, 16-ounce, wide-mouth (7)
- Measuring cups and spoons
- Mixing bowl
- Skillet
- Storage containers (3)

## STEP-BY-STEP PREP

**1.** Heat the oven to 375°F and follow the directions for Baked Boneless Chicken Thighs (page 80).

**2.** Bring a large pot of water to a boil and prep the Hard-boiled Eggs (page 82).

**3.** Heat a skillet over medium heat and follow step 1 of the Taco Salad (page 61).

**4.** While the ground beef and chicken are cooking, prep the Cauliflower Rice (page 84) for the Chicken Drumsticks and Cauliflower Rice (page 62).

**5.** Check on the chicken thighs in the oven and continue to cook the ground beef until browned. Remove both when cooked and let cool.

| | BREAKFAST | LUNCH | DINNER |
|---|---|---|---|
| DAY 1 | Fat Coffee or intermittent fasting | Chicken Caesar Salad | Chicken Drumsticks and Cauliflower Rice |
| DAY 2 | Fat Coffee or intermittent fasting | Chicken Caesar Salad | Taco Salad |
| DAY 3 | Fat Coffee or intermittent fasting | Chicken Drumsticks and Cauliflower Rice | Chicken Caesar Salad |
| DAY 4 | Fat Coffee or intermittent fasting | Chicken Caesar Salad | Taco Salad |
| DAY 5 | Fat Coffee or intermittent fasting | Taco Salad | Chicken Drumsticks and Cauliflower Rice |

6.   Prep the ingredients of the Chicken Caesar Salad (page 60) and the Taco Salad (page 61) and set aside. Prep the Caesar Dressing (page 88) for the chicken salad.

7.   Using the same skillet you used for the beef, follow steps 4 through 7 for cooking the Chicken Drumsticks (page 62).

8.   While the chicken is cooking, start to assemble the salads. Complete steps 1 and 2 of the Chicken Caesar Salad (page 60) and step 2 of the Taco Salad (page 61).

9.   When the drumsticks are done cooking, transfer them to a plate and set aside. Using the same skillet, prepare the cauliflower rice, steps 1 through 3 of Chicken Drumsticks and Cauliflower Rice (page 62).

10.   Once cool, evenly divide the rice and drumsticks into 4 storage containers and refrigerate.

# CHICKEN CAESAR SALAD | MAKES 4 SERVINGS

PREP TIME: 10 minutes

COOK TIME: 0 minutes (with precooked chicken and eggs on hand) or 30 minutes (if cooking chicken and eggs)

I was interviewed by Aaron Day on the FatForWeightLoss podcast and was asked, "What is the one keto food you can't stomach?" That would be anchovies. My husband eats them as snacks, and I just haven't been able to make that commitment yet. If it's a true Caesar salad, the dressing is made with anchovies, and the salad is topped with them as well. Even though I'm not a fan of eating anchovies themselves, I sneak anchovy paste into my homemade Caesar Dressing (page 88), and I love the depth of flavor they add.

¾ cup Caesar Dressing (page 88)

1 cup grape tomatoes

½ cup thinly sliced red onion

4 Hard-boiled Eggs (page 82), sliced

½ cup grated Parmesan cheese

2 cups chopped Baked Boneless Chicken Thighs (page 80)

1 romaine lettuce head, chopped

1.　Into each of 4 mason jars, place 3 tablespoons of dressing in the bottom.

2.　Next, add the tomatoes, onion, eggs, cheese, and chicken and top with the chopped lettuce. To serve, shake until combined.

**Storage:** Place the airtight jars in the refrigerator for up to 4 days.

**INGREDIENT TIP:** Ideally, making dressing from scratch is the way to go, but when grabbing a jar from the store is more realistic for you, keep an eye out for sugar and carbs. They both can be very sneaky. Please always check labels and serving sizes. This will soon become second nature for you. No more shopping the "fat-free" labels; instead stick to the dressings with the lowest number of ingredients.

**MAKE IT VEGETARIAN:** Skip the chicken and add extra avocado or eggs.

Per Serving: Calories: 586; Total Fat: 50g; Protein: 33g; Total Carbs: 8g; Net Carbs: 6g; Fiber: 2g; Sodium: 658mg

**Macros: 77% Fat; 22% Protein; 1% Carbs**

# TACO SALAD

**MAKES 3 SERVINGS**

PREP TIME: 10 minutes    COOK TIME: 10 minutes

Cabbage is one of my favorites to use in salads because of its great crunch. To save time, look for shredded cabbage in the bagged salad section of your local grocery store. When shopping for low-carb salsa, I usually look for the one with the lowest carb content in the deli section, no more than 5 grams of carbs per serving.

1 pound ground beef

¼ cup taco seasoning

½ cup beef broth

¾ cup low-carb salsa

¾ cup sour cream

1 cup grape tomatoes

1 (16-ounce) can sliced
  black olives

¾ cup shredded
  Cheddar cheese

1 cabbage head, shredded

2 limes, cut into wedges

1.   In a large skillet over medium heat, cook the beef until browned, 7 to 10 minutes. Add the taco seasoning and broth, and let simmer until thickened, about 3 to 5 minutes. Before assembling the salad, let the ground beef cool completely.

2.   Into 3 mason jars, divide the salsa first, then the sour cream, tomatoes, olives, cheese, ground beef, cabbage, and lime wedges. To serve, squeeze the lime wedges to release their juice, then remove them and shake the salad until combined.

**Storage**: Place the airtight jars in the refrigerator for up to 4 days.

**STORAGE TIP:** If you aren't using mason jars in this recipe (because you are already using them for the Chicken Caesar Salad), for this prep, feel free to use anything you have on hand. I would recommend keeping the sour cream and salsa stored in a separate container, unless you are using a wider container that would allow them to be stored on the side.

**SUBSTITUTION TIP:** If you want to skip prepping the beef for this recipe, feel free to add a few servings of shredded Baked Boneless Chicken Thighs (page 80) to replace it. Save even more time and buy a rotisserie chicken to use instead.

Per Serving: Calories: 931; Total Fat: 65g; Protein: 57g; Total Carbs: 34g; Net Carbs: 22g; Fiber: 12g; Sodium: 2,617mg

**Macros: 63% Fat; 24% Protein; 13% Carbs**

# CHICKEN DRUMSTICKS AND CAULIFLOWER RICE

**MAKES 3 SERVINGS**

PREP TIME: 5 minutes   COOK TIME: 30 minutes

This is one of the very first recipes I wrote and one of my family's favorites still to this day. If cauliflower isn't frequently used at your house, it needs to be! It's the perfect substitute for those high-carb veggies when living a low-carb lifestyle. It can be enjoyed mashed, roasted, boiled, or in rice form.

1 yellow onion, chopped

4 tablespoons (½ stick) salted butter, divided

3 cups uncooked Cauliflower Rice (page 84)

½ cup heavy (whipping) cream or full-fat coconut milk

½ cup shredded Cheddar cheese

Salt

Freshly ground black pepper

6 chicken drumsticks

1 tablespoon onion powder

1 tablespoon garlic salt

1. In a large skillet over medium heat, sauté the onion and 2 tablespoons of butter until the onion becomes translucent, about 5 minutes.

2. Add the cauliflower and continue to cook for 5 minutes.

3. Add the cream and cheese, and season with salt and pepper. Stir until the cheese is melted, about 2 to 3 minutes. Transfer to a serving dish and cover to keep warm.

4. In the same skillet, melt the remaining 2 tablespoons of butter over medium heat.

5. Season the drumsticks with the onion powder, garlic salt, and pepper.

6. Cook the drumsticks over medium heat for 15 minutes, turning frequently, until the skin is golden brown and the chicken is cooked through or has reached an internal temperature of 165°F.

7. Into each of 3 storage containers, place 1 cup of cauliflower rice and 2 chicken drumsticks.

**Storage:** Place the airtight containers in the refrigerator for 5 days or freeze for 3 months. To thaw, refrigerate overnight. Reheat in the microwave for 1 to 2 minutes or in a 375°F oven for 8 to 10 minutes.

**SUBSTITUTION TIP:** Try switching this recipe up by substituting your favorite kind of cheese, such as pepper Jack, for the Cheddar cheese. I am always drawn to whatever is on sale.

Per Serving: Calories: 502; Total Fat: 35g; Protein: 34g; Total Carbs: 15g; Net Carbs: 10g; Fiber: 5g; Sodium: 739mg

**Macros: 63% Fat; 27% Protein; 10% Carbs**

# MAINTENANCE WEEK 2

## SHOPPING LIST

### PANTRY

- Apple cider vinegar
- Beef broth (1 [14.5-ounce] can)
- Black pepper, ground
- Coconut oil
- Chili powder
- Cumin, ground
- Erythritol
- Extra-virgin olive oil
- Garlic salt
- Green chiles, diced (1 [4-ounce] can)
- Ketchup, no added sugar
- Pecans
- Pork rinds (½ cup)
- Salt
- Tomatoes, diced (1 [15-ounce] can)
- Tomato paste (1 [6-ounce] can)
- Walnuts
- Worcestershire sauce
- Yellow mustard, prepared

### PRODUCE

- Bell pepper, red (1)
- Broccoli florets (6 ounces)
- Celery (4 stalks)
- Green beans (1 pound)
- Mixed greens (5 ounces)
- Raspberries (1 pint)
- Scallions (3)
- Spinach (4 ounces)

### PROTEIN

- Bacon (8 ounces)
- Beef, ground (1 pound)
- Eggs, large (9)
- Pork, ground (8 ounces)
- Salmon (4 [4- to 6-ounce] fillets)
- Sausage, bulk (1 pound)

### DAIRY

- Cheddar cheese, shredded (½ cup or 2 ounces)
- Feta cheese, crumbled (1 cup or 4 ounces)
- Heavy (whipping) cream (1 pint)
- Parmesan cheese, grated (¼ cup or 1 ounce)
- Sour cream (optional)

## EQUIPMENT

- Baking sheet
- Chef's knife
- Cutting board
- Measuring cups and spoons
- Mixing bowls
- Skillet
- Slow cooker
- Storage containers (18)

## STEP-BY-STEP PREP

1. Preheat the oven to 400°F and follow steps 1 through 5 of the Sheet Pan Meat Loaf with Green Beans (page 69). Wash and reuse the bowl for the Breakfast Frittata (page 67).

2. In a cast-iron skillet, prepare the meats for the Low-Carb Chili (page 73). First, cook the ground beef, remove from the pan, and set aside. Next, cook the diced bacon, remove from the pan, and set aside. Finally, cook the sausage for both the chili and the frittata.

| | BREAKFAST | LUNCH | DINNER |
|---|---|---|---|
| **DAY 1** | Breakfast Frittata | Glazed Balsamic Salmon Salad | Sheet Pan Meat Loaf with Green Beans |
| **DAY 2** | Breakfast Frittata | Glazed Balsamic Salmon Salad | Low-Carb Chili |
| **DAY 3** | Breakfast Frittata | Low-Carb Chili | Glazed Balsamic Salmon Salad |
| **DAY 4** | Breakfast Frittata | Low-Carb Chili | Sheet Pan Meat Loaf with Green Beans |
| **DAY 5** | Breakfast Frittata | Sheet Pan Meat Loaf with Green Beans | Low-Carb Chili |

3.  Prepare the fresh ingredients in the frittata as well as the celery for the chili. Set aside.

4.  Check on the meat loaf and when done, remove from the oven and let cool. Reduce the oven temperature to 375°F for the frittata.

5.  Follow steps 1 and 2 of the Low-Carb Chili (page 73).

6.  Using the same skillet you used to prep the meats, follow steps 3 through 6 for the Breakfast Frittata (page 67).

7.  Bring a large pot of water and a dash of salt to a boil. Add the fresh green beans to the boiling water and cook for 3 to 4 minutes. Drain the beans and shock them in a bowl of ice water to stop the cooking process. Drain and follow step 6 of the meat loaf recipe. Add a slab of butter to the top of the beans in each container.

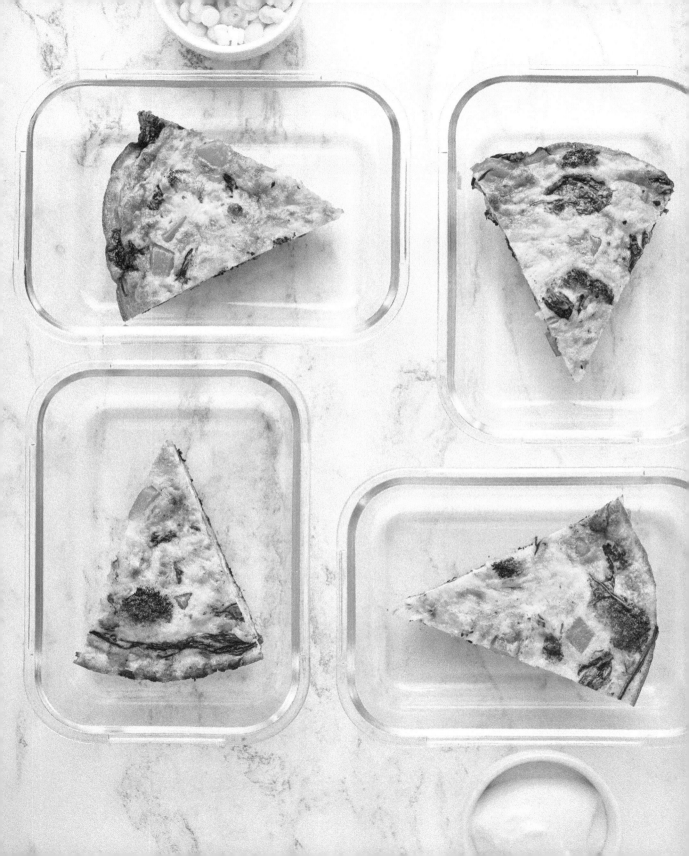

# BREAKFAST FRITTATA

**MAKES 5 SERVINGS**

PREP TIME: 10 minutes　　COOK TIME: 30 minutes

Frittatas are a great way to enjoy fluffy eggs jam-packed with healthy fats and proteins. As with the Ham and Cheese Breakfast Muffins (page 26), you can get super creative with what you put in your frittatas, so you really can't go wrong. I love cooking my protein in a cast-iron skillet so I can take advantage of the fat from the protein that coats the skillet for the vegetables and egg mixture. Talk about a crispy egg crust!

8 ounces ground sausage

1 cup chopped
　broccoli florets

1 red bell pepper, chopped

2 cups fresh spinach

8 large eggs, beaten

2 tablespoons heavy
　(whipping) cream

Salt

Freshly ground black pepper

½ cup shredded Cheddar
　cheese, divided

3 scallions, both white and
　green parts, sliced thinly

Sour cream, for serving

1.　Preheat the oven to 375°F.

2.　Heat a large cast-iron skillet over medium heat and cook the sausage until browned, 4 to 5 minutes. Remove the sausage from the skillet and drain all but 1 tablespoon of fat.

3.　In the skillet, cook the broccoli, bell pepper, and spinach until the spinach becomes slightly wilted, 2 to 3 minutes. Add the sausage back into the skillet.

4.　In a small bowl, whisk the eggs and cream and season with salt and pepper. Pour the egg mixture over the top of the broccoli and sausage mixture. Add ¼ cup of Cheddar cheese and stir the ingredients with a fork until well combined.

5.　Bake for 25 to 30 minutes, or until the top is lightly browned. Remove from the oven, add the remaining ¼ cup cheese, and put the skillet under the broiler until the cheese is melted and crisp.

6.　Let the frittata cool, cut into 5 wedges, and place each piece into each of 5 storage containers. To serve, top with the scallions and sour cream.

CONTINUED

**Storage:** Place the airtight containers in the refrigerator for up to 5 days or freeze for 3 months. To thaw, refrigerate overnight. Reheat in the microwave for 1 to 2 minutes or in a 350°F oven for 10 minutes.

**COOKING TIP:** A good frittata should have a custard-like texture, trembling and barely set. Play it safe and pull your frittata out 5 minutes before you think it's done.

**MAKE IT VEGETARIAN:** This is an easy meal to make vegetarian. Simply cut out the sausage and load on those veggies. Some of my favorites are asparagus, tomatoes, zucchini, and onions.

Per Serving: Calories: 392; Total Fat: 31g; Protein: 23g; Total Carbs: 6g; Net Carbs: 5g; Fiber: 1g; Sodium: 774mg

**Macros: 71% Fat; 23% Protein; 6% Carbs**

# SHEET PAN MEAT LOAF WITH GREEN BEANS

**MAKES 4 SERVINGS**

PREP TIME: 10 minutes    COOK TIME: 35 minutes

I was in shock the first time I simply formed meat loaf into a loaf shape with my hands instead of using a standard loaf pan. How had I never thought of this before? It makes so much sense. Baking meat loaf on an aluminum foil- or parchment-lined baking sheet makes for a quick cleanup and lets you get creative, adding in ingredients that you have on hand without worrying about adding to the size of the loaf. It also means that you can cook a small meat loaf for a family of two or a large one for a party. It's an easy way to prep healthy meals for the entire week.

8 ounces ground beef

8 ounces ground pork

1 large egg

½ cup crushed pork rinds

¼ cup grated
Parmesan cheese

¼ cup heavy
(whipping) cream

1 teaspoon prepared
yellow mustard

Salt

Freshly ground black pepper

¼ cup sugar-free ketchup or
tomato paste

1 tablespoon apple
cider vinegar

1 tablespoon erythritol

3 cups green beans,
blanched

**1.** Preheat the oven to 400°F and line a baking sheet with aluminum foil.

**2.** In a large bowl, combine the beef, pork, egg, pork rinds, Parmesan, cream, and mustard. Season with salt and pepper.

**3.** Form the mixture into a loaf shape on the prepared baking sheet.

**4.** In a small bowl, mix the ketchup, vinegar, and erythritol. Brush the mixture on top of the loaf.

**5.** Bake for 35 to 40 minutes, or until the internal temperature reaches 160°F.

**6.** Let cool and slice into 4 pieces.

**7.** Into each of 4 storage containers, place ¾ cup beans and 1 slice of meat loaf.

CONTINUED

**Storage:** Place the airtight containers in the refrigerator for up to 5 days or freeze for 3 months. To thaw, refrigerate overnight. Reheat in the microwave for 1 to 2 minutes or in a 350°F oven for 10 minutes.

**INGREDIENT TIP:** If you have some pork rinds left over, they will make for a great snack throughout the week.

**MAKE IT DAIRY-FREE:** This is one that is easy to make dairy free by omitting the Parmesan cheese and subbing coconut cream for the heavy (whipping) cream. Coconut cream is always a good alternative for cream.

Per Serving: Calories: 481; Total Fat: 27g; Protein: 49g; Total Carbs: 14g; Net Carbs: 10g; Fiber: 4g; Sodium: 833mg

**Macros: 51% Fat; 41% Protein; 8% Carbs**

# GLAZED BALSAMIC SALMON SALAD

**MAKES 4 SERVINGS**

PREP TIME: 20 minutes    COOK TIME: 15 minutes

I was a little apprehensive about including salmon in the preps because some people don't like it. Please feel free to swap out the salmon for another protein option, but I do hope you will try this combo at least once. Maybe I'll even turn you into a salmon lover! Berries are something you should eat sparingly, but the best part about that is that when you do indulge in them, they taste that much better.

4 (4- to 6-ounce) salmon fillets

2 tablespoons extra-virgin olive oil

Salt

Freshly ground black pepper

½ cup whole pecans

1 tablespoon coconut oil

1 tablespoon erythritol

4 cups mixed salad greens

¼ cup fresh raspberries or blueberries

¼ cup crumbled feta cheese (optional)

1.  Line a baking sheet with aluminum foil and preheat the broiler to high.

2.  Rub each fillet with olive oil and season with salt and pepper. Place on the prepared baking sheet and broil for 8 to 12 minutes, or until the salmon flakes easily with a fork.

3.  Remove the salmon from the baking sheet and set aside.

4.  Meanwhile, heat a skillet over medium heat and add the pecans, coconut oil, and erythritol. Stir constantly until the erythritol dissolves and the pecans become fragrant, 3 to 5 minutes. Remove from the skillet and set aside.

5.  In a large bowl, combine the mixed greens, berries, and feta.

6.  Into each of 4 storage containers, place 1 heaping cup of salad and top with a salmon fillet and 2 tablespoons of candied pecans.

CONTINUED

**Storage:** Place the airtight containers in the refrigerator for up to 4 days. Serve cold or, to reheat, remove the salmon and heat in the microwave for 1 to 2 minutes.

**INGREDIENT TIP:** I often buy a whole filleted side of salmon, especially if it's on sale. I cut it up into 4- to 6-ounce pieces and freeze whatever I have left to use at a later time.

**MAKE IT DAIRY-FREE:** Leave out the feta for a dairy-free version.

Per Serving: Calories: 456; Total Fat: 34g; Protein: 36g; Total Carbs: 9g; Net Carbs: 7g; Fiber: 2g; Sodium: 448mg

**Macros: 67% Fat; 32% Protein; 1% Carbs**

# LOW-CARB CHILI

**MAKES 5 SERVINGS**

PREP TIME: 25 minutes    COOK TIME: 4 to 6 hours on high or 8 to 10 hours on low

Who knew you could enjoy chili without the beans and gastro problems? This is a recipe I usually double to store the leftovers in the freezer for a later prep of a meal for the family.

8 ounces ground beef, cooked and drained

8 ounces uncured bacon, diced, cooked, and drained

8 ounces ground sausage, cooked and drained

1 cup beef broth

1 cup chopped celery

1 (15-ounce) can diced tomatoes, with their juices

1 (6-ounce) can tomato paste

1 (4-ounce) can diced green chiles

1 tablespoon Worcestershire sauce

1 tablespoon chili powder

1 tablespoon ground cumin

1 teaspoon garlic salt

1 teaspoon freshly ground black pepper

Shredded cheese, for garnish

Sour cream, for garnish

1.    In a large slow cooker, add the cooked beef, bacon, sausage, broth, celery, tomatoes and their juices, tomato paste, chiles, Worcestershire sauce, chili powder, cumin, garlic salt, and pepper. Stir until combined. Cook on high for 4 to 6 hours or on low for 8 to 10 hours.

2.    Let cool and divide into 5 storage containers. To serve, top with shredded cheese and sour cream.

**Storage:** Place the airtight containers in the refrigerator for up to 5 days or freeze for 3 months. To thaw, refrigerate overnight. To reheat, microwave 2 to 3 minutes or cook in a 350°F oven for 8 to 10 minutes.

Per Serving: Calories: 629; Total Fat: 37g; Protein: 46g; Total Carbs: 30g; Net Carbs: 20g; Fiber: 10g; Sodium: 1,679mg

**Macros: 53% Fat; 29% Protein; 18% Carbs**

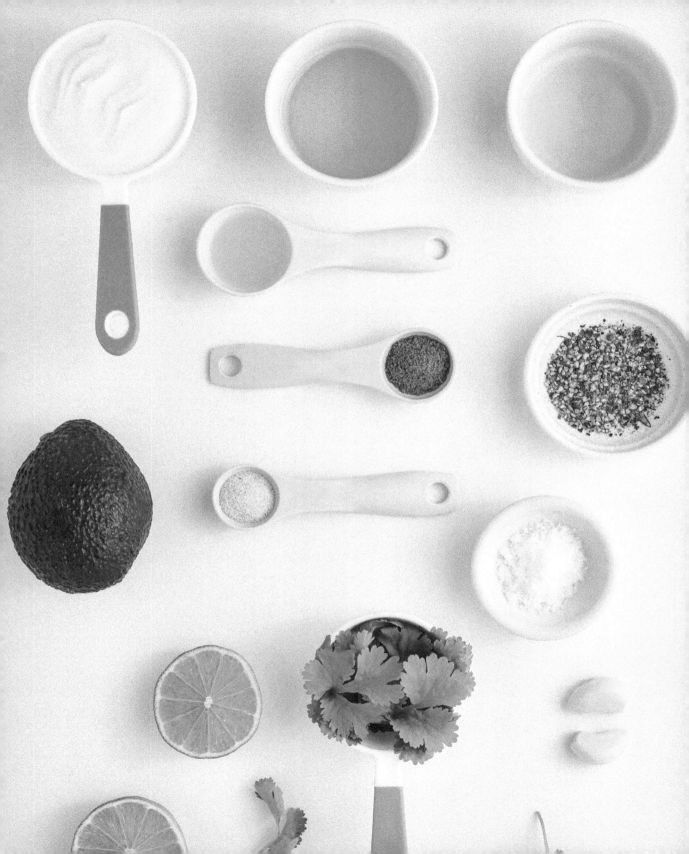

# PART THREE

# STAPLES & BONUS RECIPES

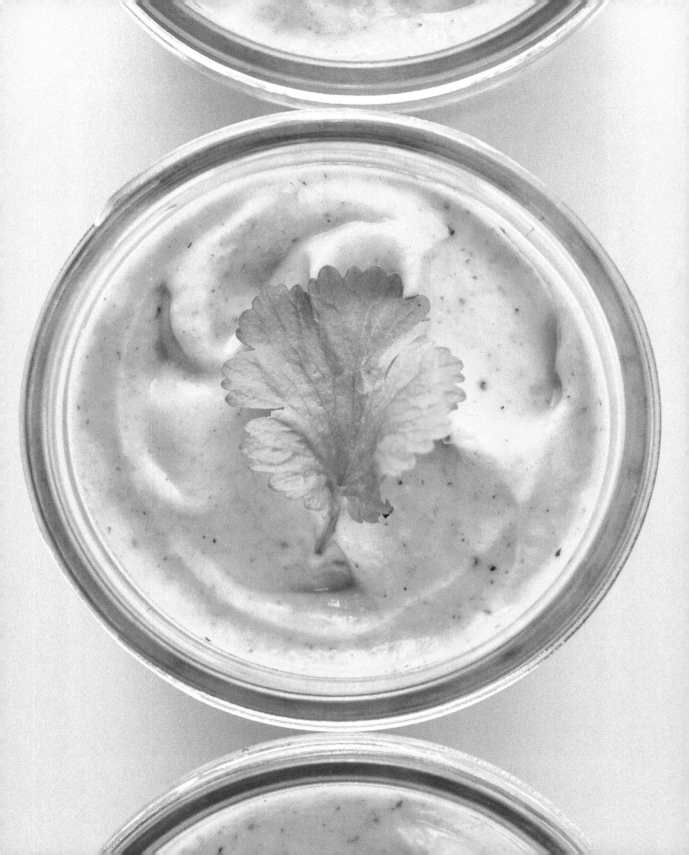

# STAPLES

« Avocado-Lime Dressing (page 91)

# FAT COFFEE

**MAKES I SERVING**

PREP TIME: 5 minutes

Fat coffee is a staple in my ketogenic lifestyle. If I don't start my mornings with a frothy cup of fat coffee, my whole day is off, including my macros. You can dress this recipe up or down, and it will keep you satisfied and full of energy for hours.

8 ounces freshly brewed coffee

1 tablespoon butter

1 tablespoon coconut oil or MCT oil

1 tablespoon heavy (whipping) cream or full-fat coconut milk

Ground cinnamon (optional)

Collagen peptides (optional)

Sea salt (optional)

MCT powder (optional)

Stevia/erythritol (optional)

1.   In a blender, combine the hot coffee, butter, coconut oil, and cream. If using, add cinnamon, collagen peptides, salt, MCT powder, and stevia. Blend for 30 seconds to 1 minute.

2.   Serve hot and embrace the fat.

**SUBSTITUTION TIP:** If you aren't a coffee drinker, you can replace the coffee in this recipe with hot tea or brewed cocoa beans. To enhance your coffee, you could also add peptides, cinnamon, cocoa powder, sweeteners, and/or sugar-free syrups to turn your hot drink into dessert.

Per Serving: Calories: 276; Total Fat: 31g; Protein: <1g; Total Carbs: <1g; Net Carbs: <1g; Fiber: <1g; Sodium: 92mg

**Macros: 99% Fat; <1% Protein; <1% Carbs**

# PERFECTLY COOKED BACON

**MAKES 6 SERVINGS**

PREP TIME: 5 minutes    COOK TIME: 15 minutes

Who would have thought you could eat bacon while dieting and living a healthy lifestyle? I used to keep bacon out of my diet because of the fat content and all the sodium. But when you live a ketogenic lifestyle, your body needs more of both. Remember that uncured, sugar-free bacon is best!

1 to 2 pounds uncured bacon

1.    Preheat the oven to 375°F. Line a baking sheet with aluminum foil.

2.    Arrange the bacon slices directly next to each other on the prepared baking sheet.

3.    Cook the bacon for 12 to 20 minutes, depending on the thickness and how crispy you like yours.

4.    Transfer the bacon to a plate lined with paper towels to drain.

**Storage:** Place in an airtight container in the refrigerator for 4 to 5 days.

**VARIATION TIP:** You can also cook bacon on the stovetop. Start with a cold skillet (cast iron preferred) and lay the bacon slices next to each other in the bottom. Cook slowly on low heat for 8 to 12 minutes, or to your desired crispness.

Per Serving: Calories: 308; Total Fat: 24g; Protein: 21g; Total Carbs: <1g; Net Carbs: <1g; Fiber: 0g; Sodium: 1,317mg

**Macros: 70% Fat; 29% Protein; <1% Carbs**

# BAKED BONELESS CHICKEN THIGHS

**MAKES 6 SERVINGS**

PREP TIME: 5 minutes    COOK TIME: 25 minutes

Not all cuts of chicken are alike as far as macronutrients go when you consider the fat content. A 6-ounce boneless, skinless chicken breast has 4 grams of fat and 38 grams of protein. A 6-ounce chicken thigh has 14 grams of fat and 39 grams of protein—and it just tastes better. When you are shopping for poultry, look for darker cuts of meat for higher fat content.

2 pounds boneless, skinless chicken thighs

1 tablespoon onion powder

1 tablespoon garlic powder

Salt

Freshly ground black pepper

**1.** Preheat the oven to 375°F. Line a baking sheet with parchment paper or aluminum foil.

**2.** Place the thighs on the prepared baking sheet and season with the onion powder, garlic powder, salt, and pepper.

**3.** Bake the chicken for 25 to 30 minutes, or until the internal temperature reaches 165°F and the juices run clear.

**4.** Let cool and slice into strips for easy use. Divide the sliced chicken between 6 storage containers.

**Storage:** Place the airtight containers in the refrigerator for up to 6 days or freeze for 3 months. To thaw, refrigerate overnight. Reheat in the microwave for 1 to 2 minutes or in a 375°F oven for 8 to 10 minutes.

> **VARIATION TIP:** If you have the time, throwing the thighs in a marinade the night (or even 30 minutes) before you bake them will totally be worth it. To make a simple chicken marinade, combine ¼ cup avocado oil, ¼ cup sesame oil, 2 tablespoons coconut aminos, 1 teaspoon ground ginger, salt, and pepper.

Per Serving: Calories: 153; Total Fat: 10g; Protein: 16g; Total Carbs: 0g; Net Carbs: 0g; Fiber: 0g; Sodium: 356mg

**Macros: 40% Fat; 60% Protein; 0% Carbs**

# HARD-BOILED EGGS

**MAKES 12 SERVINGS**

PREP TIME: 5 minutes     COOK TIME: 15 minutes

Hard-boiled eggs are a great source of fat to add to any salad, easy to eat on the go, and quick to make into keto-friendly deviled eggs. I make a batch of hard-boiled eggs at the start of the week and my family always goes through them by the end of the week.

12 large eggs, at room temperature

1.  In a large stockpot, arrange the eggs in a single layer. Add enough cold water to cover the eggs by one inch. Bring to a boil over high heat.

2.  Remove the pot from the heat and cover with a lid. Let it sit for 15 minutes.

3.  Pour out the hot water and place the eggs in a large bowl full of ice water for 30 minutes.

**Storage:** Place in an airtight container, peeled or unpeeled, and refrigerate for 7 days.

Per Serving: Calories: 63; Total Fat: 4g; Protein: 6g; Total Carbs: <1g; Net Carbs: <1g; Fiber: 0g; Sodium: 62mg

**Macros: 57% Fat; 38% Protein; 5% Carbs**

# ZUCCHINI NOODLES

**MAKES 4 SERVINGS**

PREP TIME: 20 minutes    COOK TIME: 5 minutes

A vegetable spiralizer is well worth the small investment when you go low carb. When living keto, there are so many options for rich, savory, and cheesy dressings and sauces. Replacing the starchy noodles with noodle-like, low-carb veggies leaves you feeling guilt-free and with a happy stomach. It's also a great way to get the kiddos to eat their veggies.

4 zucchini

3 tablespoons butter or extra-virgin olive oil

1 teaspoon minced garlic

Salt

Freshly ground black pepper

**1.** Cut the zucchini into noodles using a spiralizer, julienne peeler, or knife. Set the noodles aside.

**2.** In a large skillet, melt the butter over medium-high. Add the garlic and cook for 1 minute, or until it becomes translucent.

**3.** Add the zucchini noodles and toss to coat the noodles in butter. Cook for 2 to 5 minutes, or until tender. Zucchini can turn to mush very quickly, so be careful not to overcook it. The noodles should have a bit of crunch to them.

**4.** Divide the noodles evenly between 4 storage containers. (You can also divide the uncooked noodles among containers after step 1.)

**Storage**: Place the airtight containers of either cooked or uncooked zucchini noodles in the refrigerator for up to 5 days. Reheat in the microwave for 1 to 2 minutes.

Per Serving: Calories: 109; Total Fat: 9g; Protein: 3g; Total Carbs: 7g; Net Carbs: 5g; Fiber: 2g; Sodium: 372mg

**Macros: 74% Fat; 11% Protein; 15% Carbs**

# CAULIFLOWER RICE

**MAKES 4 SERVINGS**

PREP TIME: 10 minutes    COOK TIME: 10 minutes

Cauliflower is something I've really grown to love, and it's my favorite ingredient to experiment with in the kitchen. Cauliflower rice is a perfect replacement anytime a dish calls for white rice, brown rice, or couscous. Get creative with cauliflower! The options are endless and are all low carb.

**FOR RAW CAULIFLOWER RICE**

1 head cauliflower, trimmed

**FOR COOKED CAULIFLOWER RICE**

2 tablespoons butter or
extra-virgin olive oil
2 cups raw cauliflower rice
Salt
Freshly ground black pepper

**TO MAKE RAW CAULIFLOWER RICE**

1.   Wash and dry the cauliflower. Cut the head into 4 pieces, and remove any greens.

2.   With your hands, break the cauliflower apart into large florets.

3.   Fill the food processor three-quarters of the way full with florets, working in batches as needed.

4.   Process the cauliflower in 1 to 2 second pulses, until it is completely broken down and resembles rice. Raw cauliflower rice can be used in salads to replace grains.

**TO MAKE COOKED CAULIFLOWER RICE**

1.   In a large skillet with a lid, heat the butter over medium heat.

2.   Add the riced cauliflower to the skillet and season with salt and pepper.

3.   Cook, stirring until the cauliflower is coated in butter, about 1 minute.

4.   Cover the skillet with the lid and cook, stirring occasionally, until the cauliflower is tender, 5 to 8 minutes.

5.   Divide the cauliflower rice between 4 storage containers. Let cool and cover.

**Storage**: Place the airtight containers in the refrigerator for up to 5 days for an easy and quick weeknight side dish. Reheat in the microwave for 1 to 2 minutes or in a 375°F oven for 8 to 10 minutes.

**COOKING TIP:** If you don't have a food processor, try a box grater to create riced cauliflower. You can also check out your local grocery store. I see more and more stores starting to carry prepped cauliflower rice, so be sure to check your produce section.

Per Serving: Calories: 67; Total Fat: 6g; Protein: 1g; Total Carbs: 4g; Net Carbs: 2g; Fiber: 2g; Sodium: 351mg

**Macros: 80% Fat; 5% Protein; 15% Carbs**

# SPAGHETTI SQUASH

**MAKES 5 SERVINGS**

PREP TIME: 5 minutes    COOK TIME: 35 minutes

Spaghetti squash is a winter squash, but unlike other winter squashes, it's low in calories and starch. One serving of cooked spaghetti squash has 19 calories, 4 grams of carbs, and 0 grams of fiber. This makes it a great alternative to pasta and gives you the freedom to enjoy Alfredo (page 114) or Bolognese (page 45).

1 (4-pound) spaghetti squash

1.    Preheat the oven to 375°F.

2.    Cut the spaghetti squash lengthwise and remove the seeds. Place the halves, cut-side down, in a baking dish and fill the bottom with a quarter inch of water.

3.    Bake for 35 to 40 minutes, or until tender. Let cool. Use a fork to remove the spaghetti-like strands from the squash.

4.    Divide the squash between 5 storage containers.

**Storage:** Place the airtight containers in the refrigerator for up to 5 days. Reheat in the microwave for 1 to 2 minutes or in a 375°F oven for 8 to 10 minutes.

Per Serving: Calories: 19; Total Fat: <1g; Protein: <1g; Total Carbs: 4g; Net Carbs: 4g; Fiber: 0g; Sodium: 10mg

**Macros: <1% Fat; <1% Protein; 99% Carbs**

# MAYONNAISE

## MAKES ABOUT 2 CUPS

PREP TIME: 10 minutes

This recipe for mayonnaise is simple to make, can be stored for up to a week, and makes for a guilt-free addition to any dish. Incorporating mayonnaise into your meal is a great way to stay within your fat goals for the day. Before beginning this recipe, make sure the ingredients are at room temperature so that the eggs disperse evenly.

2 large egg yolks, at room temperature

1 teaspoon salt

1 teaspoon Dijon mustard

2 tablespoons freshly squeezed lemon juice

1 tablespoon apple cider vinegar or white vinegar

1½ cups extra-virgin olive oil or avocado oil

1.   In a food processor, blend the yolks, salt, mustard, lemon juice, and vinegar for about 30 seconds, or until the mixture thickens.

2.   With the food processor running on high speed, slowly drizzle the oil into the egg mixture until it thickens.

3.   Transfer to a storage container or jar.

**Storage:** Place the airtight container or jar in the refrigerator for up to a week.

**TIME-SAVING TIP:** If you don't have time to break out the food processor and throw this together (I promise it takes less than 10 minutes), look for the lowest-carb mayo at your local supermarket. I recommend the brand Primal Kitchen.

Per Serving (2 tablespoons): Calories: 188; Total Fat: 21g; Protein: <1g; Total Carbs: <1g; Net Carbs: <1g; Fiber: 0g; Sodium: 152mg

**Macros: 99% Fat; <1% Protein; <1% Carbs**

# CAESAR DRESSING

**MAKES ABOUT 1 CUP**

PREP TIME: 10 minutes

A few years ago, at a fine Italian restaurant, I ordered a beautiful Caesar salad topped with aged Parmesan cheese and whole anchovies. Until that day, I was unaware that anchovies played such an important role in Caesar salads. My point being, don't let the anchovy paste in the ingredient list scare you away from this recipe. If you have enjoyed a Caesar salad in the past, you've most likely enjoyed the flavor of anchovies as well. Just like salt and pepper, anchovy paste and Worcestershire sauce can vary according to your taste. Play around with the amounts and find a balance that satisfies your palate.

2 garlic cloves, peeled and smashed

2 large egg yolks

Juice of 1 lemon

1 teaspoon prepared yellow mustard

1 teaspoon anchovy paste

1 teaspoon Worcestershire sauce

½ cup extra-virgin olive oil or avocado oil

¼ cup grated Parmesan cheese

Salt

Freshly ground black pepper

**1.** In a blender, add the garlic, egg yolks, lemon, mustard, anchovy paste, and Worcestershire sauce. Blend for 30 seconds, or until the mixture becomes smooth.

**2.** With the blender running on medium speed, slowly drizzle the oil in until the dressing become thick and creamy.

**3.** Stir in the Parmesan cheese and season generously with salt and pepper.

**4.** Transfer to a jar or storage container and chill for at least 30 minutes before serving.

**Storage:** Place the airtight jar or container in the refrigerator for up to a week.

**INGREDIENT TIP:** Shop for anchovies and anchovy paste near the canned tuna in your grocery store.

Per Serving (2 tablespoons): Calories: 152; Total Fat: 17g; Protein: 2g; Total Carbs: 1g; Net Carbs: 1g; Fiber: <1g; Sodium: 83mg

**Macros: 99% Fat; <1% Protein; <1% Carbs**

# BALSAMIC DRESSING

**MAKES ½ CUP**

PREP TIME: 5 minutes

Balsamic dressing isn't something you have to go without when living keto. Most balsamic dressings or glazes are high in sugar, and that's why I encourage you to take the time to make your own. That way, you can use your preferred low-carb sweetener.

½ tablespoon butter

2 garlic cloves, minced

¼ cup balsamic vinegar

⅓ cup extra-virgin olive oil

3 tablespoons Dijon mustard

1 tablespoon erythritol

Salt

Freshly ground black pepper

1.   In a skillet over medium heat, combine the butter and garlic. Cook, stirring occasionally, until the garlic is browned, 3 to 5 minutes.

2.   Remove from the heat, drain off the butter, and add the garlic to a small bowl.

3.   In the same bowl, add the balsamic vinegar, oil, mustard, and erythritol. Season with salt and pepper. Whisk together until combined.

4.   Transfer to a storage container or jar.

**Storage:** Place the airtight container or jar in the refrigerator for up to a week.

Per Serving (1 tablespoon): Calories: 93; Total Fat: 10g; Protein: <1g; Total Carbs: 3g; Net Carbs: 3g; Fiber: <1g; Sodium: 189mg

**Macros: 97% Fat; <1% Protein; 2% Carbs**

# DAIRY-FREE RANCH DRESSING

## MAKES ABOUT 1½ CUPS

PREP TIME: 10 minutes

This ranch dressing is super versatile and easy to make. It's a great addition to any salad, a perfect topping for steamed or roasted vegetables, and even works as a marinade. If you are short on time or in a pickle, look for the ranch dressing with the lowest carbs in the refrigerated produce section of your grocery store. I love the vegan ranch made by Follow Your Heart. It's high in fat, dairy-free, and very low in carbs.

1 cup Mayonnaise (page 87)

½ cup canned full-fat coconut milk

2 garlic cloves, finely minced

1 tablespoon freshly squeezed lemon juice

1 tablespoon apple cider vinegar

2 tablespoons chopped fresh Italian parsley

Salt

Freshly ground black pepper

1.  In a blender, combine the Mayonnaise, coconut milk, garlic, lemon juice, vinegar, and parsley. Season with salt and pepper.

2.  Blend on high for 1 to 2 minutes, or until smooth.

3.  Transfer to a jar or storage container and chill for at least 1 hour before serving.

**Storage:** Place the airtight jar or container in the refrigerator for up to a week.

Per Serving (2 tablespoons): Calories: 135; Total Fat: 12g; Protein: <1g; Total Carbs: 7g; Net Carbs: 7g; Fiber: <1g; Sodium: 317mg

**Macros: 80% Fat; <1% Protein; 19% Carbs**

# AVOCADO-LIME DRESSING

**MAKES 1 CUP**

PREP TIME: 10 minutes

The biggest challenge in creating a keto meal prep book was not being able to use fresh avocado since, by the second day, you would have a very brown avocado on top of your salad or lettuce wrap. This dressing is a great way to take advantage of the multiple benefits of incorporating avocado into your high-fat lifestyle. Many keto followers aren't fond of avocados due to their texture, and this way you can sneak it in through a tasty dressing.

1 medium avocado, halved, pitted, and peeled

1 bunch cilantro, leaves chopped

2 garlic cloves, peeled

½ cup sour cream

3 tablespoons extra-virgin olive oil

1 tablespoon apple cider vinegar

1 tablespoon freshly squeezed lime juice

1 teaspoon salt

½ teaspoon garlic powder

½ teaspoon ground cumin

½ teaspoon freshly ground black pepper

1 jalapeño pepper, seeded and minced (optional)

1. In a food processor or blender, combine the avocado, cilantro, garlic, sour cream, oil, vinegar, lime juice, salt, garlic powder, cumin, pepper, and jalapeño, if using.

2. Process until smooth.

3. Add water or cream if the dressing is too thick, or add a little more avocado to thicken up a too-runny dressing.

4. Transfer to a jar or storage container.

**Storage:** Place the airtight jar or container in the refrigerator for up to 4 days.

**INGREDIENT TIP:** The brand Primal Kitchen makes great alternative marinades and dressings. Their products are made with avocado oil, and I haven't tried one I don't like!

Per Serving: Calories: 131; Total Fat: 13g; Protein: 1g; Total Carbs: 4g; Net Carbs: 2g; Fiber: 2g; Sodium: 301mg

**Macros: 89% Fat; 3% Protein; 8% Carbs**

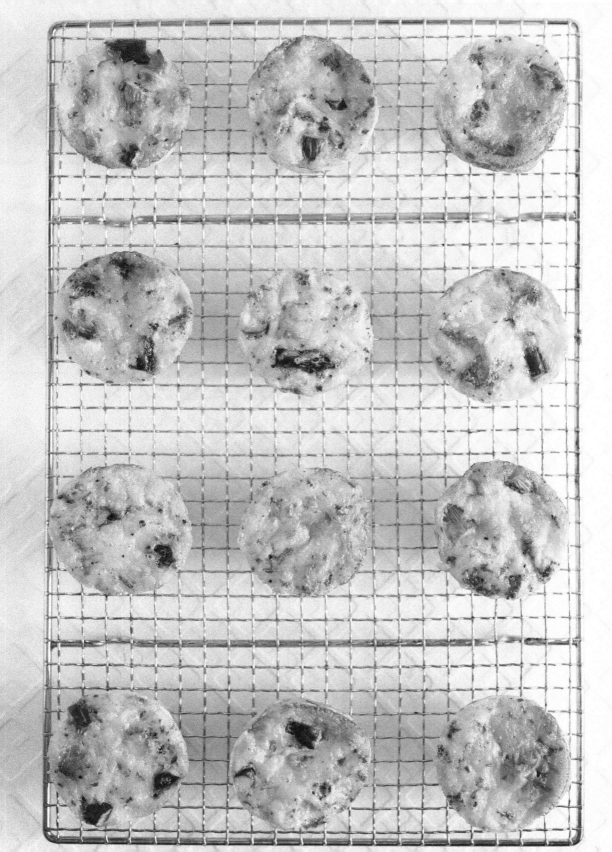

# BREAKFAST

« Bacon-Asparagus Breakfast Muffins (page 98)

# COCONUT FLOUR PANCAKES

**MAKES 6 SERVINGS**

PREP TIME: 10 minutes    COOK TIME: 15 minutes

Coconut flour has a great texture for pancakes, and these don't taste super coconutty. While you may be tempted to make the batter ahead and cook the pancakes fresh, I don't recommend it. Cook these pancakes before you store them. As time passes, coconut flour soaks up more and more liquid, making the batter difficult to work with if it sits. Top with a sugar-free, low-carb pancake syrup or with a few berries and whipped cream sweetened with a pinch of erythritol.

1 cup melted unsalted butter or coconut oil

1 cup heavy (whipping) cream or full-fat coconut milk

8 large eggs, beaten

1 teaspoon vanilla extract

1 cup coconut flour

1 tablespoon erythritol

2 teaspoons baking soda

Pinch salt

1. In a medium bowl, whisk together the butter, cream, eggs, and vanilla.

2. In a large bowl, whisk together the coconut flour, erythritol, baking soda, and salt.

3. Add the wet ingredients to the dry and mix until just combined.

4. Heat a nonstick griddle or skillet over medium-high. Brush with a little melted butter or coconut oil.

5. In ¼-cup portions, spoon the batter onto the hot griddle. Cook until bubbles form on top, about 2 minutes.

6. Flip with a spatula. Cook 2 to 3 minutes more, or until lightly browned on the bottom.

7. Into each of 6 storage containers, place 3 pancakes.

**Storage:** Place the airtight containers in the refrigerator for up to 5 days or in the freezer for up to 6 months. To thaw, refrigerate overnight. Reheat in the microwave for 1 minute or until warm, or in a 350°F oven for 5 to 10 minutes.

Per Serving: Calories: 518; Total Fat: 40g; Protein: 13g; Total Carbs: 31g; Fiber: 16g; Net Carbs: 15g; Sodium: 646mg

**Macros: 70% Fat; 10% Protein; 20% Carbs**

# OMELET-STUFFED BAKED BELL PEPPERS

**MAKES 4 SERVINGS**

PREP TIME: 10 minutes     COOK TIME: 55 minutes

These peppers make a perfect breakfast on the go because they store well and reheat in the microwave. Use any color bell pepper you like. Be sure to remove any seeds or fibrous ribs from the peppers to help reduce bitterness and heat.

2 red bell peppers, halved lengthwise, seeds and ribs removed

½ pound bulk Italian sausage

4 ounces mushrooms, sliced

8 large eggs, beaten

¼ cup heavy (whipping) cream

1 teaspoon Italian seasoning

½ teaspoon salt

⅛ teaspoon freshly ground black pepper

Pinch red pepper flakes

½ cup grated Parmesan cheese

1. Preheat the oven to 400°F.

2. Place the peppers on a rimmed baking sheet with the cut sides up. Bake in the oven for 5 minutes to soften.

3. Meanwhile, in a large nonstick skillet, heat the sausage over medium-high heat, crumbling with a spoon, until it is browned, about 5 minutes.

4. Add the mushrooms and cook, stirring occasionally, until soft, another 5 minutes. Cool slightly.

5. In a bowl, whisk together the eggs, cream, Italian seasoning, salt, pepper, and red pepper flakes.

6. Fold in the cooled sausage and mushrooms.

7. Pour the mixture into the pepper halves. Sprinkle with the cheese.

8. Return to the oven. Cook until the eggs are set and the cheese is browned, about 40 minutes. Let cool.

9. Into each of 4 storage containers, place 1 stuffed pepper half.

CONTINUED

**Storage:** Place the airtight containers in the refrigerator for up to 5 days or freeze for up to 6 months. To thaw, refrigerate overnight. Reheat in the microwave for 1 to 2 minutes or in a 400°F oven for about 30 minutes.

**SUBSTITUTION TIP:** Replace the Italian sausage with ½ pound of bacon or pancetta, fried and crumbled.

Per Serving: Calories: 459; Total Fat: 34g; Protein: 33g; Total Carbs: 7g; Net Carbs: 6g; Fiber: 1g; Sodium: 1,048mg

**Macros: 67% Fat; 29% Protein; 4% Carbs**

# TEX-MEX SCRAMBLE

**MAKES 4 SERVINGS**

PREP TIME: 10 minutes    COOK TIME: 15 minutes

If you like a spicy breakfast, then this is perfect for you. Garnish, if desired, with a little bit of sour cream to cool it down or your favorite guacamole. It cooks quickly, stores well, and reheats easily.

8 ounces bulk chorizo

6 scallions, both white and green parts, chopped

1 jalapeño pepper, seeded and minced

2 garlic cloves, minced

8 large eggs, beaten

½ cup grated Cheddar cheese

1.  In a large nonstick skillet, cook the chorizo over medium-high heat, crumbling with a spatula as you cook, until it is browned, about 5 minutes.

2.  Add the scallions and jalapeño and cook, stirring occasionally, until softened, about 3 minutes more.

3.  Add the garlic and cook, stirring constantly, for 30 seconds.

4.  Add the eggs to the pan.

5.  Cook, scrambling, until the eggs are set, about 3 minutes.

6.  Sprinkle with the cheese. Stir once to combine on the heat.

7.  Divide the scramble evenly between 4 storage containers.

**Storage:** Place the airtight containers in the refrigerator for up to 3 days or freeze for up to 6 months. To thaw, refrigerate overnight. Reheat in the microwave on high for 1 to 2 minutes.

Per Serving: Calories: 508; Total Fat: 40g; Saturated Fat: 17g; Protein: 32g; Total Carbs: 5g; Fiber: <1g; Sugar: 2g; Sodium: 1,002mg

**Macros: 71% Fat; 25% Protein; 4% Carbs**

# BACON-ASPARAGUS BREAKFAST MUFFINS

**MAKES 6 SERVINGS**

PREP TIME: 10 minutes     COOK TIME: 25 minutes

If you only have a 6-cup muffin tin, then you can halve this recipe. Silicone muffin tins are especially good for making breakfast egg muffins because they release so easily. Feel free to vary the ham or veggies in this recipe.

Coconut oil, butter, or extra-virgin olive oil, for greasing

4 tablespoons (½ stick) unsalted butter

8 ounces bacon, chopped

½ onion, chopped

1 pound asparagus, trimmed and cut into bite-size pieces

1 cup shredded Gruyère or Swiss cheese

10 large eggs, beaten

¼ cup heavy (whipping) cream

1 teaspoon Dijon mustard

1 teaspoon dried rosemary

½ teaspoon salt

⅛ teaspoon freshly ground black pepper

1. Preheat the oven to 375°F. Grease a 12-cup muffin tin.

2. In a large nonstick skillet, heat the butter over medium-high until it bubbles. Add the bacon and cook until it browns, about 5 minutes.

3. Add the onion and asparagus and cook, stirring occasionally, until the vegetables are tender, about 5 minutes.

4. Spoon into the prepared muffin cups.

5. Sprinkle with the cheese.

6. In a large bowl, whisk together the eggs, cream, mustard, rosemary, salt, and pepper.

7. Pour over the vegetables and cheese in the muffin cups.

8. Bake in the preheated oven until the eggs are set, 12 to 15 minutes. Let cool slightly and remove the muffins from the tin. Into each of 6 storage containers, place 2 muffins.

**Storage:** Place the airtight containers in the refrigerator for 3 days or freeze for up to 6 months. To thaw, refrigerate overnight. Reheat for 1 to 2 minutes in the microwave or in a 375°F oven for about 10 minutes.

Per Serving: Calories: 411; Total Fat: 31g; Protein: 27g; Total Carbs: 7g; Net Carbs: 5g; Fiber: 2g; Sodium: 900mg

**Macros: 68% Fat; 26% Protein; 6% Carbs**

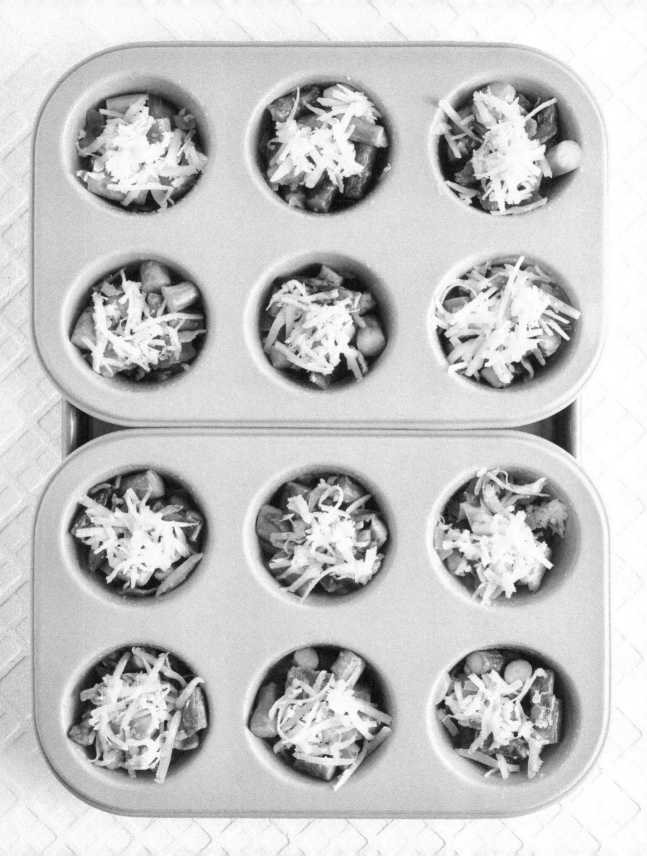

# BACON AND EGG CUPS WITH AVOCADO HOLLANDAISE

**MAKES 6 SERVINGS**

PREP TIME: 10 minutes    COOK TIME: 20 minutes

If you like eggs Benedict, this recipe offers a quick, easy keto variation. Normally hollandaise sauce can be tricky and requires precise timing on the stove. This version is made quickly in the blender using creamy avocado and lots of citrus to keep it from browning.

6 slices bacon

6 large eggs

Freshly ground black pepper

1 avocado, halved, pitted, and peeled

½ cup hot water

Juice and zest of 1 lemon

½ teaspoon salt

Pinch cayenne pepper

¼ cup extra-virgin olive oil

1. Preheat the oven to 400°F.

2. Line 6 cups of a nonstick muffin tin with the bacon slices. Season with pepper.

3. Bake for 10 minutes.

4. Remove from the oven and carefully crack 1 egg into each cup.

5. Return to the oven and bake until the eggs are set, about 10 minutes more.

6. Meanwhile, in a blender, combine the avocado, hot water, lemon juice and zest, salt, and cayenne. Blend until smooth, pausing once or twice to scrape down the sides of the blender.

7. With the blender running, drizzle in the olive oil in a thin stream until it is fully incorporated. Divide into 6 single-serving storage containers.

8. When the egg cups are done cooking, remove them from the muffin tin.

9. Into each of 6 storage containers, place 1 egg cup. To serve, drizzle with the hollandaise sauce.

**Storage:** Place the airtight containers of hollandaise sauce and egg cups separately in the refrigerator. The hollandaise will only keep for a few days in the refrigerator, so it's best made on demand, but the egg cups will keep in the refrigerator for about 4 days.

**SUBSTITUTION TIP:** You can also use Canadian bacon, which is the classic meat used with eggs Benedict.

**INGREDIENT TIP:** I recommend using a creamy Hass avocado for this recipe. You can tell Hass avocados by their bumpy, green-to-black skin.

Per Serving: Calories: 428; Total Fat: 42g; Protein: 9g; Total Carbs: 5g; Net Carbs: 2g Fiber: 3g; Sodium: 608mg

**Macros: 88% Fat; 9% Protein; 3% Carbs**

# CARAMELIZED ONION FRITTATA

**MAKES 4 SERVINGS**

PREP TIME: 10 minutes    COOK TIME: 35 minutes

A *frittata* is a very keto, cost-effective Italian dish—and my go-to meal when I have some veggies I need to use and some leftover protein. It also happens to make for a quick and easy meal prep option. Traditionally, frittatas are round because they are baked in a cast iron skillet, but if you're using a baking dish instead, then square ones are just as good.

¼ cup avocado oil

1 yellow onion, thinly sliced, or ½ recipe of Caramelized Onions (page 130)

1 teaspoon dried thyme

½ teaspoon salt

⅛ teaspoon freshly ground black pepper

8 large eggs, beaten

1. Preheat the broiler on high and adjust the rack to the top position.

2. In a large ovenproof skillet, heat the oil over medium-high until it shimmers.

3. Add the onions, thyme, salt, and pepper. Stir once or twice and turn the burner down to medium-low.

4. Cook, stirring occasionally, until the onions are deeply browned, about 30 minutes. Spread them in an even layer on the bottom of the skillet.

5. Pour the beaten eggs carefully over the onions. Cook until the eggs are set on the edges. Use a spatula to pull the set edges away from the side of the pan, tilt the pan, and allow the uncooked eggs to run into the spaces you've cleared. Cook until set again about 20 to 35 minutes.

6. Transfer to the broiler and cook until the eggs are puffy and brown on top, 3 to 5 minutes.

7. Let cool and cut into 4 wedges.

8. Into each of 4 storage containers, place 1 wedge of frittata.

**Storage:** Place the airtight containers in the refrigerator for up to 5 days or in the freezer for up to 6 months. To thaw, refrigerate overnight. Reheat for 1 to 2 minutes in the microwave or in a 375°F oven for 5 to 10 minutes.

> **VARIATION TIP:** If dairy-free isn't necessary, you can add ½ cup of grated Swiss cheese or Asiago cheese to the top of the frittata just before you put it under the broiler.

Per Serving: Calories: 156; Total Fat: 11g; Protein: 12g; Total Carbs: 4g; Net Carbs: 11g; Fiber: 1g; Sodium: 359mg

**Macros: 63% Fat; 31% Protein; 6% Carbs**

# BREAKFAST PIZZA FRITTATA

**MAKES 4 SERVINGS**

PREP TIME: 10 minutes    COOK TIME: 10 minutes

Remember the days of eating cold pizza for breakfast? This frittata is the grown-up version of cold pizza—warm, fragrant, and gooey. Feel free to switch toppings to make a pizza with the flavors you love.

2 tablespoons unsalted butter

8 ounces cubed pancetta

½ onion, finely chopped

1 cup sliced mushrooms

8 large eggs, beaten

¼ cup heavy (whipping) cream

1 teaspoon dried oregano

Pinch red pepper flakes

½ cup shredded mozzarella cheese

8 cherry tomatoes, halved

1.  Preheat the broiler on high and adjust the rack to the top position.

2.  In a large ovenproof skillet, heat the butter over medium-high heat until it bubbles. Add the pancetta and cook, stirring occasionally, until it starts to brown, 3 to 5 minutes.

3.  Add the onion and mushrooms and cook, stirring occasionally, until the veggies are soft, about 3 minutes more. Spread in an even layer in the bottom of the pan.

4.  Whisk together the eggs, cream, oregano, and red pepper flakes. Pour into the hot pan. Cook without stirring, allowing the eggs to set around the edges. Using a spatula, pull back the set edges, tilt the pan, and allow the uncooked eggs to run into the openings. Cook until the edges are set again about 3 minutes.

5.  Sprinkle the cheese over the eggs and top with the tomatoes. Put under the preheated broiler until the cheese melts and browns slightly, 3 to 5 minutes.

6.  Let cool slightly and cut into 4 wedges.

7.  Into each of 4 storage containers, place 1 wedge of frittata.

**Storage:** Place the airtight containers in the refrigerator for up to 5 days or in the freezer for up to 6 months. To thaw, refrigerate overnight. Reheat for 1 to 2 minutes in the microwave or in a 375°F oven for 5 to 10 minutes.

**SUBSTITUTION TIP:** Replace the pancetta with chopped Canadian bacon or chopped pepperoni. If you do, instead of precooking the meat before adding the veggies, cook the meat and veggies together until the vegetables are soft, about 4 minutes. You can also replace the mozzarella cheese with Parmesan cheese.

Per Serving: Calories: 644; Total Fat: 47g; Protein: 43g; Total Carbs: 14g; Net Carbs: 10g; Fiber: 4g; Sodium: 1,660mg

**Macros: 66% Fat; 27% Protein; 7% Carbs**

# SAUSAGE, EGG, AND CHEESE CASSEROLE

**MAKES 12 SERVINGS**

PREP TIME: 10 minutes    COOK TIME: 1 hour and 10 minutes

This recipe makes a lot, and it freezes well, which means it's a perfect prep meal. With a few simple variations, you can change the flavors and ingredients enough that you have plenty of variety. Make a few different flavor variations, freeze them, and then choose what sounds good to you each morning.

1 pound bulk
  breakfast sausage

1 onion, chopped

9 large eggs, beaten

1 cup heavy
  (whipping) cream

½ teaspoon salt

⅛ teaspoon freshly ground
  black pepper

1 cup shredded Swiss cheese

1. Preheat the oven to 350°F. Grease a 9-by-13-inch baking dish.

2. Heat a large nonstick skillet to medium-high.

3. Add the sausage and cook, crumbling with a spoon or a spatula, until it is browned, about 5 minutes.

4. Add the onion and cook until it softens, 2 to 3 minutes more. Remove from the heat and set aside.

5. While the sausage cools, in a large bowl beat the eggs, cream, salt, and pepper.

6. Fold in the sausage and cheese.

7. Spread in a single layer in the prepared baking dish.

8. Bake until set, about 1 hour.

9. Cool slightly before slicing into 12 pieces.

10. Into each of 12 storage containers, place 1 piece.

**Storage:** Place the airtight containers in the refrigerator for up to 5 days or in the freezer for up to 6 months. Reheat from frozen in a 350°F oven for about 20 minutes, or thaw in the refrigerator overnight and reheat in the microwave for 1 to 2 minutes.

**SUBSTITUTION TIP:** You can also make a spicy Tex-Mex version of this by replacing the sausage with bulk chorizo and the Swiss cheese with shredded pepper Jack.

Per Serving: Calories: 285; Total Fat: 23g; Protein: 17g; Total Carbs: 2g; Net Carbs: 2g; Fiber: <1g; Sodium: 448mg

**Macros: 72% Fat; 24% Protein; 4% Carbs**

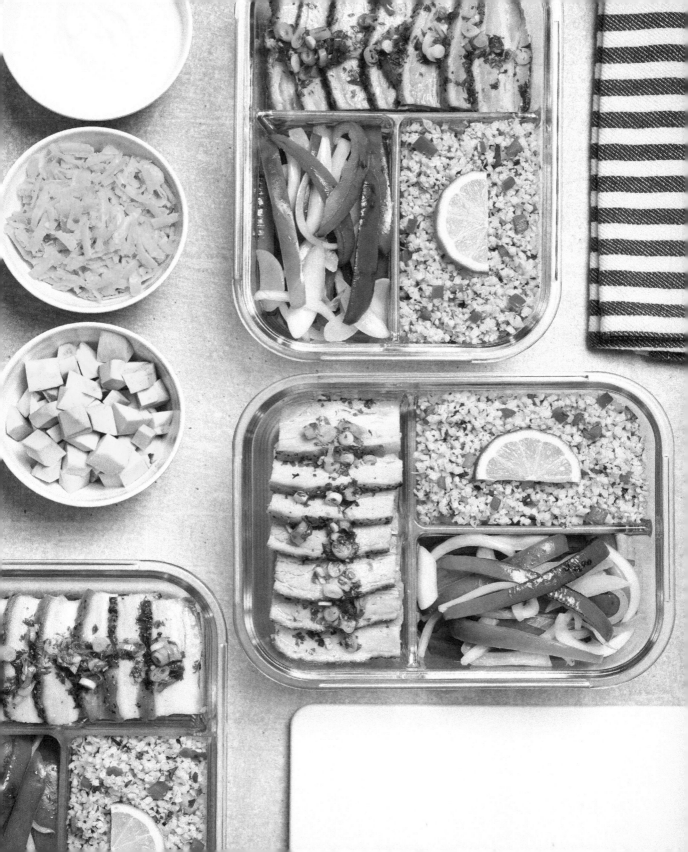

# LUNCH AND DINNER

◀◀ Pork Burrito Bowls (page 118)

# SALMON SALAD

**MAKES 4 SERVINGS**

PREP TIME: 10 minutes

Salmon salad makes a great take-it-with-you meal. Eat it alone or rolled up in lettuce, or spread it over a bed of your favorite greens for a quick and tasty lunch or dinner.

8 ounces flaked salmon (fresh or canned)

3 scallions, both white and green parts, finely chopped

3 dill pickles, finely chopped

½ cup Mayonnaise (page 87)

3 tablespoons extra-virgin olive oil

1 teaspoon Dijon mustard

Juice and zest of 1 lemon

1 teaspoon dried dill

⅛ teaspoon freshly ground black pepper

1. In a large bowl, combine the salmon, scallions, and pickles.

2. In a small bowl, whisk together the mayonnaise, oil, mustard, lemon juice and zest, dill, and pepper.

3. Mix the dressing into the salmon mixture.

4. Divide the salad between 4 storage containers.

**Storage:** This doesn't freeze well, but it will keep in the refrigerator in the airtight containers for up to 5 days.

**SUBSTITUTION TIP:** You can also use canned tuna or cooked fresh baby shrimp for this salad.

Per Serving: Calories: 446; Total Fat: 31g; Protein: 34g; Total Carbs: 11g; Net Carbs: 9g; Fiber: 2g; Sodium: 1,086mg

**Macros: 62% Fat; 30% Protein; 8% Carbs**

# CHOPPED CHICKEN SALAD WITH MUSTARD VINAIGRETTE

**MAKES 4 SERVINGS**

PREP TIME: 15 minutes

Using grocery store premade rotisserie chicken makes this recipe no-cook and super quick. Feel free to add additional veggies or cheese to the salad depending on your flavor preferences—but make sure if you do add veggies that they aren't starchy.

1 pound dark meat and skin from a rotisserie chicken, chopped

2 Hard-boiled Eggs (page 82), peeled and chopped

½ cup sliced black olives

1 red bell pepper, seeded and chopped

1 (14-ounce) can artichoke hearts, drained and chopped

8 cherry tomatoes, quartered

2 tablespoons Dijon mustard

½ cup extra-virgin olive oil

3 tablespoons apple cider vinegar

1 tablespoon minced shallot

½ teaspoon salt

⅛ teaspoon freshly ground black pepper

Pinch red pepper flakes

**1.** In a large bowl, combine the chicken, eggs, olives, bell pepper, artichoke hearts, and cherry tomatoes.

**2.** In a small bowl, whisk together the mustard, oil, vinegar, shallot, salt, pepper, and red pepper flakes.

**3.** Divide the chicken salad between 4 storage containers, and divide the vinaigrette between 4 single-serve storage containers. To serve, toss the dressing with the salad.

**Storage:** The dressing won't freeze well, but it will keep in the refrigerator, covered, for a week. The covered salad will keep in the refrigerator for about 5 days.

Per Serving: Calories: 499; Total Fat: 40g; Protein: 22g; Total Carbs: 18g; Net Carbs: 12g; Fiber: 6g; Sugar: 9g; Sodium: 596mg

**Macros: 72% Fat; 18% Protein; 10% Carbs**

# CREAM OF MUSHROOM SOUP

**MAKES 4 SERVINGS**

PREP TIME: 15 minutes, plus 1 hour steeping time   COOK TIME: 10 minutes

Dried porcini mushrooms give a deep mushroom flavor to this tasty soup. If you can't find dried porcini mushrooms, then use any type of dried mushrooms you can find.

1 (2-ounce) package dried porcini mushrooms

3 cups sodium-free vegetable broth or chicken broth

4 tablespoons (½ stick) unsalted butter

1 shallot, finely chopped

1 pound cremini mushrooms, sliced

½ cup sherry or dry white wine

1 teaspoon dried thyme

½ teaspoon salt

⅛ teaspoon freshly ground black pepper

1½ cups heavy (whipping) cream

1. In a medium pot, bring the dried porcini mushrooms and vegetable broth to a simmer. Remove from the heat and let steep for at least an hour. The longer you allow it to steep, the more mushroom flavor the broth will have.

2. Strain the mushrooms from the broth. Chop the mushrooms and reserve the broth.

3. In a large pot, heat the butter over medium-high until it shimmers. Add the shallot and cremini mushrooms and cook, stirring occasionally, until the mushrooms are deeply browned, 5 to 7 minutes.

4. Add the sherry and cook, stirring, for 1 minute.

5. Add the reserved broth and chopped mushrooms, thyme, salt, and pepper. Bring to a simmer.

6. Stir in the cream. Cook, stirring constantly, until the soup begins to simmer, about 5 minutes.

7. Into each of 4 storage containers, place 1½ cups of the soup.

**Storage:** Place the airtight containers in the refrigerator for up to 5 days or freeze for up to 6 months. To thaw, refrigerate overnight. Reheat on the stovetop over medium-high heat for a few minutes, until warm.

**COOKING TIP:** You can use this recipe for other dishes, such as Cheesy Green Bean Casserole (page 133), or enjoy it as a soup.

Per Serving: Calories: 355; Total Fat: 29g; Protein: 8g; Total Carbs: 17g; Net Carbs: 13g; Fiber: 4g; Sugar: 5g; Sodium: 355mg

**Macros: 74% Fat; 9% Protein; 17% Carbs**

# ARROZ CON POLLO

**MAKES 4 SERVINGS**

PREP TIME: 15 minutes     COOK TIME: 20 minutes

One of the great things about Tex-Mex flavors is that you can jazz them up with extras like chopped avocados or a tablespoon of sour cream for additional flavor. This version of arroz con pollo, made with riced cauliflower, is mildly spicy and utterly delicious.

¼ cup avocado oil

1 pound boneless, skinless chicken thighs, chopped

1 onion, chopped

8 ounces mushrooms, sliced

1 (14-ounce) can crushed tomatoes, with their juices

1 tablespoon chili powder

1 teaspoon dried oregano

1 teaspoon ground cumin

1 teaspoon garlic powder

½ teaspoon salt

Pinch cayenne pepper

2 cups uncooked Cauliflower Rice (page 84)

1 cup shredded Monterey Jack cheese

½ cup sour cream, for garnish

**1.** In a large nonstick skillet, heat the avocado oil over medium-high until it shimmers.

**2.** Add the chicken and cook, stirring occasionally, until it is browned, about 5 minutes. Using a slotted spoon, remove the chicken from the oil and set it aside.

**3.** Add the onion and mushrooms to the skillet. Cook, stirring occasionally, until the vegetables are browned, about 5 minutes.

**4.** Return the chicken to the skillet with the vegetables, adding any juices that have collected on the plate.

**5.** Add the tomatoes and their juices, chili powder, oregano, cumin, garlic powder, salt, and cayenne. Bring to a simmer, stirring.

**6.** Add the cauliflower. Cook, stirring occasionally, for 5 minutes.

**7.** Add the cheese. Cook, stirring, just until the cheese melts and mixes in, about 2 minutes more.

**8.** Into 4 containers, divide the chicken and cauliflower rice. To serve, garnish with the sour cream.

**Storage:** Store the airtight containers in the refrigerator for up to 5 days or in the freezer for up to 6 months. To thaw, refrigerate overnight. Reheat in the microwave for 1 to 2 minutes.

Per Serving: Calories: 513; Total Fat: 35g; Protein: 31g; Total Carbs: 20g; Net Carbs: 13g; Fiber: 7g; Sodium: 687mg

**Macros: 61% Fat; 24% Protein; 15% Carbs**

# FETTUCCINE ALFREDO WITH MUSHROOMS AND PANCETTA

**MAKES 6 SERVINGS**

PREP TIME: 10 minutes    COOK TIME: 20 minutes

The sauce is everything in this recipe: creamy, delicious, and it keeps well. Store the "noodles" separately from the sauce. You can buy premade zucchini noodles at the grocery store, but it's really easy to make them by using a vegetable peeler to peel long, wide, ribbon-shaped strips from a zucchini.

- 4 tablespoons extra-virgin olive oil, divided
- 6 ounces pancetta, cubed
- 2 tablespoons minced shallot
- 8 ounces mushrooms, sliced
- 4 zucchini, cut into ribbons with a vegetable peeler
- 3 garlic cloves, minced
- 8 ounces cream cheese
- 8 tablespoons (1 stick) unsalted butter
- ½ cup heavy (whipping) cream
- 1 cup grated Parmesan cheese
- ⅛ teaspoon freshly ground black pepper

1.  In a large skillet, heat 2 tablespoons of oil over medium-high heat until it shimmers. Add the pancetta and cook until it's browned, about 5 minutes. Using a slotted spoon, remove it from the oil and set it aside on a platter.

2.  Add the remaining 2 tablespoons of oil to the pan. Add the shallot and mushrooms to the skillet. Cook, stirring occasionally, until browned, about 5 minutes. Add the zucchini and cook, stirring occasionally, for about 3 minutes more, until the zucchini is just tender. Add the garlic and cook, stirring constantly, for 30 seconds. Return the pancetta to the pan and cook for 30 seconds more to rewarm the pancetta.

3.  While the vegetables cook, in a medium pot, heat the cream cheese, butter, cream, Parmesan, and pepper over medium-low heat, whisking as it melts to combine it completely. Cook, whisking, until heated through, about 5 minutes.

4.  Into 4 divided containers, place the vegetables on one side and the sauce on the other. To serve, mix the vegetables and sauce together.

**Storage:** Place the airtight containers in the refrigerator for up to 4 days or in the freezer for up to 6 months. To thaw, refrigerate overnight. Reheat the sauce and noodles separately before combining. Reheat in the microwave for 1 to 2 minutes or on the stovetop over medium-high heat until warm. You may need to add a little milk to adjust the consistency.

**MAKE IT VEGETARIAN:** Omit the pancetta to make this vegetarian. You can also add a pinch of red pepper flakes to the veggies for heat.

Per Serving: Calories: 691; Total Fat: 62g; Protein: 29g; Total Carbs: 10g; Net Carbs: 8g; Fiber: 2g; Sodium: 1,246mg

**Macros: 80% Fat; 17% Protein; 3% Carbs**

# TUNA CASSEROLE

**MAKES 9 SERVINGS**

**PREP TIME:** 20 minutes    **COOK TIME:** 1 hour and 10 minutes

This simple tuna casserole uses the Cream of Mushroom Soup (page 112). Zucchini pieces replace noodles, but you won't miss the noodles at all because this casserole is loaded with flavor.

¼ cup avocado oil

1 onion, chopped

2 zucchini, sliced

3 garlic cloves, minced

1 recipe Cream of Mushroom Soup (page 112), cooled

Zest of 1 lemon

1 teaspoon dried dill

1 tablespoon Dijon mustard

1 pound oil-packed tuna, drained

1 cup shredded Cheddar cheese

**1.** Preheat the oven to 350°F.

**2.** In a large nonstick skillet, heat the oil over medium-high heat until it shimmers. Add the onion and zucchini and cook, stirring occasionally, until the veggies start to soften, about 5 minutes.

**3.** Add the garlic and cook, stirring constantly, for 30 seconds. Remove from the heat and cool.

**4.** In a large bowl, combine the cream of mushroom soup, lemon zest, dill, and mustard. Whisk until smooth. Add the cooled vegetables, tuna, and cheese. Mix to combine.

**5.** Spread into a 9-by-13-inch baking dish. Bake until bubbling, about 1 hour. Let cool.

**6.** Divide the casserole between 9 storage containers.

**Storage:** Place the airtight containers in the refrigerator for up to 3 days or freeze for up to 6 months. To thaw, refrigerate overnight. Reheat in the microwave for 1 to 2 minutes or in a 375°F oven for 15 to 20 minutes.

Per Serving: Calories: 761; Total Fat: 59g; Protein: 53g; Total Carbs: 12g; Net Carbs: 9g; Fiber: 3g; Sodium: 473mg

**Macros: 70% Fat; 28% Protein; 2% Carbs**

# CHEESY CHICKEN AND MUSHROOM CASSEROLE

**MAKES 8 SERVINGS**

PREP TIME: 20 minutes    COOK TIME: 1 hour and 15 minutes

This recipe is creamy, filling, delicious, and it's easy to prep. It freezes well (up to six months in individual servings) or lasts about three days in the fridge. You can also make this in an Instant Pot®—pressure cook on high for 20 minutes.

8 bone-in chicken thighs

1 pound button mushrooms, halved

1 (8-ounce) bag frozen pearl onions

1 recipe Cream of Mushroom Soup (page 112), cooled

1 cup shredded Cheddar cheese

1. Preheat the oven to 350°F.

2. In a 9-by-13-inch baking dish, arrange the chicken thighs, mushrooms, and onions so they are well mixed but spread throughout the pan.

3. In a bowl, stir the soup and cheese together. Pour over the chicken, mushrooms, and onions.

4. Bake, covered with aluminum foil, for 1 hour and 15 minutes, or until the chicken is cooked through and its juices run clear. Let cool.

5. Divide the casserole between 8 storage containers.

**Storage:** Place the airtight containers in the refrigerator for up to 3 days or freeze for up to 6 months. To thaw, refrigerate overnight. Reheat for 1 to 2 minutes in the microwave or in a 375°F oven for 20 to 30 minutes.

**VARIATION TIP:** Serve this with the sauce spooned over cooked Cauliflower Rice (page 84) if you wish, or over the Cauliflower Mash (page 131).

Per Serving: Calories: 609; Total Fat: 56g; Protein: 25g; Total Carbs: 11g; Net Carbs: 9g; Fiber: 2g; Sodium: 383mg

**Macros: 83% Fat; 16% Protein; 1% Carbs**

# PORK BURRITO BOWLS

**MAKES 4 SERVINGS**

PREP TIME: 15 minutes, plus 4 to 8 hours marinating time     COOK TIME: 20 minutes

Burrito bowls store and reheat well—and they're delicious. If possible, make the marinade in the morning and let the meat marinate in it for at least eight hours to really allow the flavors to penetrate. Cook the meat and peppers at dinnertime.

½ cup avocado oil, divided

1 bunch fresh cilantro, leaves chopped

Juice of 3 limes

1 jalapeño pepper, minced

½ teaspoon salt

6 garlic cloves, minced

6 scallions, both white and green parts, finely minced

1 pound pork belly

1 onion, sliced

1 green bell pepper, thinly sliced

2 cups cooked Cauliflower Rice (page 84)

1 cup shredded Cheddar cheese

½ cup sour cream

1 avocado, halved, pitted, and chopped

1. In a medium bowl, whisk together ¼ cup of the oil, the cilantro, lime juice, jalapeño, salt, garlic, and scallions. Set aside 2 tablespoons of the mixture.

2. Add the remaining mixture to a large zip-top bag and add the pork belly. Coat the meat with the marinade, seal the bag, and refrigerate for 4 to 8 hours.

3. In a large skillet, heat the remaining ¼ cup of oil on over medium-high heat until it shimmers.

4. Remove the meat from the marinade and wipe away any excess. Cook it in the hot oil until it reaches an internal temperature of 145°F, about 5 minutes per side. Set aside on a platter, tented with foil, to rest.

5. In the same skillet, add the onion and bell pepper. Cook, stirring occasionally, until the veggies are soft, about 5 minutes.

6. Slice the meat thinly against the grain and return it to the pan. Add the reserved 2 tablespoons of marinade. Cook, stirring, for 2 minutes, or until the meat and veggies are coated with the marinade.

7. Into 4 storage containers, divide the sliced pork and vegetables, and into each of 4 separate storage containers, place ½ cup cauliflower rice. To serve, mix the meat, veggies, and cauliflower rice together and top with the cheese, sour cream, and avocado.

**Storage:** Place the airtight containers in the refrigerator for up to 5 days. Reheat in the microwave for 1 to 2 minutes.

**COOKING TIP:** If you have a food processor or blender, make the marinade by pulsing the avocado oil, cilantro, lime juice, jalapeño, salt, garlic, and scallions in the food processor or blender until it resembles pesto.

Per Serving: Calories: 528; Total Fat: 35g; Protein: 41g; Total Carbs: 18g; Net Carbs: 12g; Fiber: 6g; Sodium: 474mg

**Macros: 60% Fat; 31% Protein; 9% Carbs**

# SLOW COOKER BEEF STEW

**MAKES 8 SERVINGS**

PREP TIME: 15 minutes    COOK TIME: 4 hours on high or 8 hours on low

This is a recipe that will keep well in the freezer and lends itself to really large batches, so if you have a large slow cooker, you can double it. It's also super easy—put it in the slow cooker in the morning and let it go for the day. You'll come home in the evening to a really nice-smelling house and some delicious, hearty food.

1½ pounds chuck roast or stew meat, cut into cubes

2 red onions, roughly chopped

1 pound button mushrooms, halved or quartered (depending on size)

1 (8-ounce) bag frozen pearl onions

4 celery stalks, roughly chopped

1 cup dry red wine (such as Cabernet Sauvignon or Syrah)

2 teaspoons garlic powder

1 tablespoon Dijon mustard

1 teaspoon dried thyme

1 teaspoon dried rosemary

1 teaspoon salt

¼ teaspoon freshly ground black pepper

1.    In a slow cooker, combine the beef, red onions, mushrooms, pearl onions, celery, wine, garlic powder, mustard, thyme, rosemary, salt, and pepper. Stir to combine.

2.    Cover and cook on high for 4 hours or on low for 8 hours. Let cool.

3.    Into each of 8 storage containers, place 1½ cups of stew.

**Storage:** Place the airtight containers in the refrigerator for up to 5 days or freeze for up to 6 months. To thaw, refrigerate overnight. Reheat in the microwave for 1 to 2 minutes or on the stovetop over medium-high, stirring occasionally, about 5 minutes. You may need to add a little broth to adjust the thickness.

Per Serving: Calories: 933; Total Fat: 66g; Protein: 69g; Total Carbs: 7g; Net Carbs: 6g; Fiber: 1g; Sodium: 433mg

**Macros: 64% Fat; 30% Protein; 6% Carbs**

# SLOW COOKER PORK CHILI

**MAKES 8 SERVINGS**

PREP TIME: 15 minutes    COOK TIME: 4 hours on high or 8 hours on low

This is a really easy chili recipe, and it freezes well. Plus, you can make big batches. If you have a large slow cooker, double the recipe and use it for meals for months to come. You can also use country-style pork ribs (with bones removed) for this recipe. Just cube them before you add them to the slow cooker.

2 pounds boneless pork shoulder, cut into cubes

1 onion, chopped

3 tablespoons chili powder

1 teaspoon ground coriander

1 teaspoon garlic powder

1 teaspoon ground cumin

1 teaspoon salt

1 cup shredded Cheddar cheese

1 cup sour cream

1.    In a large slow cooker, combine the pork shoulder, onion, chili powder, coriander, garlic powder, cumin, and salt.

2.    Stir to mix. Cover and cook on high for 4 hours or on low for 8 hours. Let cool.

3.    Into each of 8 storage containers, place 1½ cups of chili. To serve, garnish with the cheese and sour cream.

**Storage:** Place the airtight containers in the refrigerator for up to 5 days or freeze for up to 6 months. To thaw, refrigerate overnight. Reheat in the microwave for 1 to 2 minutes or on the stovetop over medium-high heat, stirring occasionally. You may need to add a little broth to adjust the thickness.

**COOKING TIP:** The pork is usually fatty enough that you don't need water. However, if the pork seems lean, add up to a ½ cup of water to the slow cooker.

Per Serving: Calories: 466; Total Fat: 36g; Protein: 31g; Total Carbs: 5g; Net Carbs: 4g; Fiber: 1g; Sodium: 268mg

**Macros: 70% Fat; 27% Protein; 3% Carbs**

# PORK STIR-FRY

**MAKES 6 SERVINGS**

PREP TIME: 15 minutes    COOK TIME: 10 minutes

Stir-fries are great because they cook up so quickly, and they're quite easy to vary. This version has all of the tasty flavors of a pork pot sticker minus the high-carb outer dumpling, so if you like a good pot sticker, you'll enjoy this stir-fry.

3 tablespoons coconut oil

1 pound ground pork

6 scallions, both white and green parts, sliced

2 cups shredded green cabbage or bagged coleslaw mix

1 tablespoon grated peeled fresh ginger

3 garlic cloves, minced

Juice of 2 limes

1 tablespoon low-sodium soy sauce

½ teaspoon sesame oil

½ teaspoon chili oil

1.   In a large skillet, heat the coconut oil over medium-high heat until it shimmers.

2.   Add the pork and cook, stirring, until it just starts to brown, about 5 minutes.

3.   Add the scallions, cabbage, and ginger. Cook, stirring, until the vegetables soften, about 3 minutes more.

4.   Add the garlic and cook, stirring constantly, for about 30 seconds.

5.   Add the lime juice, soy sauce, sesame oil, and chili oil. Cook for 1 to 2 minutes, or until heated through.

6.   Divide the stir-fry between 6 storage containers.

**Storage:** Place the airtight containers in the refrigerator for up to 3 days or freeze for up to 6 months. To thaw, refrigerate overnight. Reheat in the microwave for 1 to 2 minutes.

**VARIATION TIP:** If you have fresh cilantro, stir in some chopped cilantro at the end of cooking or use as a garnish. You can also garnish with chopped peanuts, cashews, or sesame seeds.

Per Serving: Calories: 698; Total Fat: 50g; Protein: 54g; Total Carbs: 5g; Net Carbs: 4g; Fiber: 1g; Sodium: 367mg

**Macros: 64% Fat; 31% Protein; 5% Carbs**

# MEATY LASAGNA

**MAKES 12 SERVINGS**

PREP TIME: 20 minutes    COOK TIME: 1 hour and 15 minutes

This recipe is hearty and very filling. It's great to make for a crowd, but it also keeps very well in the refrigerator or freezer, so it's the perfect meal prep recipe. It has a few steps and takes a little time, but the payoff in the sheer volume of food you have for the coming weeks makes it totally worth it.

¼ cup avocado oil

1 shallot, minced

6 garlic cloves, minced

2 (14-ounce) cans crushed tomatoes (1 can drained, the other with juices reserved)

1 teaspoon Italian seasoning

1 pound bulk Italian sausage

1 (7-ounce) container prepared pesto

1 (15-ounce) container whole-milk ricotta cheese

16 ounces sliced salami

3 cups shredded mozzarella cheese, divided

1. Preheat the oven to 350°F.

2. In a large skillet, heat the oil over medium-high heat until it shimmers.

3. Add the shallot and cook, stirring, for 2 minutes. Add the garlic and cook, stirring constantly, for 30 seconds.

4. Add the tomatoes, along with the juices of 1 can, and the Italian seasoning. Bring to a simmer. Simmer, stirring occasionally, for 5 minutes.

5. As the sauce simmers, in another large skillet, heat the Italian sausage over medium-high heat, crumbling with a spoon until it is browned, about 5 minutes. Remove from the heat and set aside.

6. In a small bowl, mix the pesto and ricotta.

7. Spread about a ½ cup of the sauce on the bottom of a 9-by-13-inch baking dish.

8. Layer a single layer of salami in the pan over the sauce, and spread with a thin layer of the pesto and ricotta mixture. Sprinkle with 1 cup of the shredded cheese. Spread about ¼ to ½ cup more of the sauce over the top, add another layer of salami and another layer of the ricotta mixture, and another cup of the shredded cheese.

**9.** Spread a final layer of salami over the top of the shredded cheese and cover with the remaining sauce. Sprinkle with the remaining cup of shredded cheese.

**10.** Put the pan on a rimmed baking sheet to catch any drips and place it in the oven. Bake for 1 hour. Allow to cool slightly before slicing into 12 pieces.

**11.** Into each of 12 storage containers, place 1 piece of lasagna.

**Storage:** Place the airtight containers in the refrigerator for up to 5 days or freeze for up to 6 months. Reheat from frozen in a 350°F oven for about 45 minutes, or thaw in the refrigerator overnight and reheat in the microwave for 1 to 2 minutes.

Per Serving: Calories: 554; Total Fat: 43g; Protein: 29g; Total Carbs: 11g; Net Carbs: 9g; Fiber: 2g; Sodium: 1,296mg

**Macros: 71% Fat; 20% Protein; 9% Carbs**

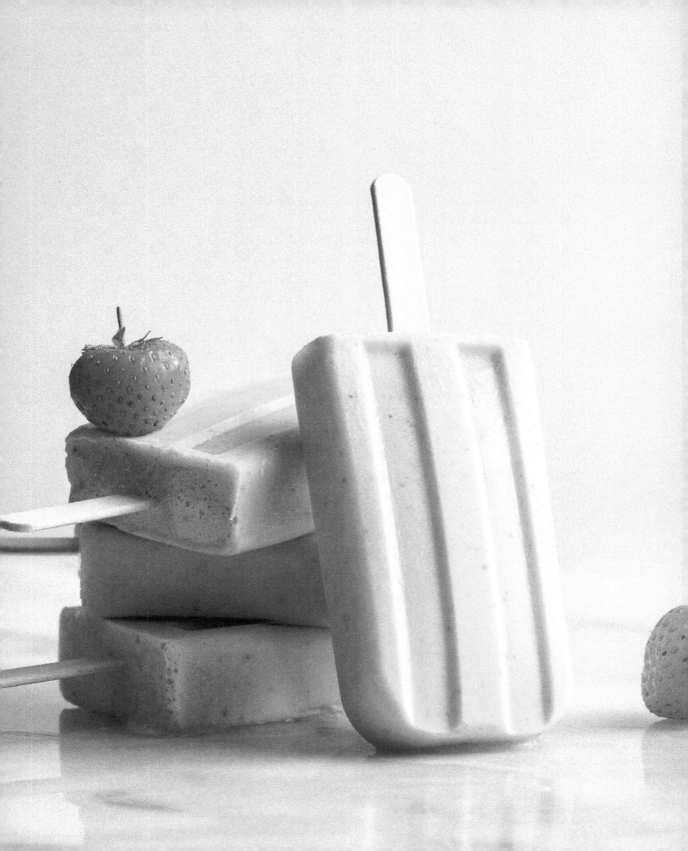

# VEGETABLES AND SNACKS

◀◀ Blended Strawberry-Coconut Ice Pops (page 140)

# SPICY COLESLAW

**MAKES 4 SERVINGS**

PREP TIME: 5 minutes

This coleslaw is super easy to make and take. It has a vinegar-based dressing instead of a creamy one, but it's still really flavorful. It's best to store the vinaigrette separately from the coleslaw to keep the cabbage crunchy.

4 cups shredded green cabbage or bagged coleslaw mix

6 scallions, both white and green parts, finely chopped

1 bunch fresh cilantro, leaves chopped

¼ cup apple cider vinegar

½ cup avocado oil

Juice of 1 lime

½ teaspoon sriracha or ¼ teaspoon chili oil

½ teaspoon Chinese hot mustard

1 tablespoon sesame seeds

1 garlic clove, minced

1 teaspoon grated peeled fresh ginger

½ teaspoon salt

**1.** In a large bowl, combine the cabbage, scallions, and cilantro, tossing to mix.

**2.** In a small bowl, whisk together the vinegar, oil, lime juice, sriracha, mustard, sesame seeds, garlic, ginger, and salt.

**3.** Into each of 4 storage containers, place 1 cup of the coleslaw. Into each of 4 single-serving containers, place 3 tablespoons of the dressing. To serve, toss the coleslaw with the dressing.

**Storage:** Place the airtight containers in the refrigerator. The dressing will keep in the refrigerator for up to a week and the slaw for up to 5 days. Do not freeze.

Per Serving: Calories: 103; Total Fat: 7g; Protein: 2g; Total Carbs: 11g; Net Carbs: 7g; Fiber: 4g; Sodium: 290mg

**Macros: 61% Fat; 8% Protein; 31% Carbs**

# CAPRESE CHOPPED SALAD

**MAKES 4 SERVINGS**

PREP TIME: 10 minutes

A simple Caprese salad is a beautiful thing. This version is chopped so it will store well. It tastes best when tomatoes and basil are in season, especially if you can find heirloom tomatoes. It's also really delicious with fresh mozzarella if you can find it.

3 large heirloom tomatoes, chopped

1 bunch fresh basil, leaves chopped

12 ounces fresh mozzarella cheese, chopped

¼ cup extra-virgin olive oil

½ teaspoon salt

⅛ teaspoon freshly ground black pepper

In a large bowl, combine the tomatoes, basil, mozzarella, oil, salt, and pepper. Toss to mix. Divide the salad between 4 storage containers.

**Storage:** Place the airtight containers in the refrigerator for up to 3 days. Do not freeze.

Per Serving: Calories: 373; Total Fat: 28g; Protein: 25g; Total Carbs: 8g; Net Carbs: 6g; Fiber: 2g; Sodium: 751mg

**Macros: 68% Fat; 27% Protein; 5% Carbs**

# CARAMELIZED ONIONS

**MAKES ABOUT 2 CUPS**

PREP TIME: 10 minutes    COOK TIME: 20 minutes

While you don't necessarily eat caramelized onions on their own (although they're great on a steak), they make a flavorful add-in to casseroles, soups, dips, and many of the recipes in this book. Here's how to make a big batch ahead of time.

¼ cup avocado oil

4 onions, sliced thinly

1 teaspoon salt

1. In a large nonstick skillet, heat the oil over medium-high heat until it shimmers.

2. Reduce the heat to medium-low and add the onions and salt.

3. Cook, stirring occasionally, until the onions are deeply caramelized, 20 to 30 minutes.

4. Into each of 4 storage containers, place a ½-cup serving.

**Storage:** Place the airtight containers in the refrigerator for up to 5 days or freeze for up to 6 months. To thaw, refrigerate overnight.

Per Serving: Calories: 63; Total Fat: 2g; Protein: 1g; Total Carbs: 11g; Net Carbs: 8g; Fiber: 3g; Sodium: 473mg

**Macros: 29% Fat; 6% Protein; 65% Carbs**

# CAULIFLOWER MASH

**MAKES 4 SERVINGS**

PREP TIME: 20 minutes    COOK TIME: 10 minutes

If you haven't tried it yet, then you may be surprised at what a tasty substitute mashed cauliflower makes for mashed potatoes. Serve this as a side dish, on its own, or as a side for any dinner with a sauce, such as the Baked Boneless Chicken Thighs (page 80). This recipe easily doubles or triples.

1 cauliflower head

¼ cup unsalted melted butter

¼ cup heavy (whipping) cream

½ teaspoon salt

⅛ teaspoon freshly ground black pepper

1. Break the cauliflower into florets and put them in a large pot covered with water. Over medium-high heat, bring the water to a boil.

2. Boil until the cauliflower florets are soft, about 10 minutes.

3. Drain. Using a potato masher, mash the cauliflower. Stir in the butter, cream, salt, and pepper.

4. Divide the cauliflower mash between 4 storage containers.

**Storage:** Place the airtight containers in the refrigerator for up to 5 days or freeze for up to 6 months. To thaw, refrigerate overnight. Reheat in the microwave for 1 to 2 minutes or on the stovetop over medium-high heat, stirring occasionally. You may need to add a little milk to adjust the thickness.

**VARIATION TIP:** Add flavor by stirring in Caramelized Onions (page 130) or boiling a few garlic cloves with the cauliflower and then mashing them with the cauliflower.

Per Serving: Calories: 143; Total Fat: 14g; Protein: 3g; Total Carbs: 5g; Net Carbs: 3g; Fiber: 2g; Sodium: 262mg

**Macros: 88% Fat; 8% Protein; 4% Carbs**

# ROASTED BRUSSELS SPROUTS WITH BACON

**MAKES 4 SERVINGS**

PREP TIME: 10 minutes    COOK TIME: 20 minutes

Roasting Brussels sprouts brings out the rich caramel notes in the sprouts, and bacon is always a welcome addition for smokiness and flavor. Make a batch of these on the weekend and then reheat them in the microwave during the week.

¼ cup avocado oil

1½ pounds Brussels sprouts, halved lengthwise

4 ounces bacon, chopped

½ teaspoon salt

⅛ teaspoon freshly ground black pepper

1.  Preheat the oven to 400°F.

2.  In a large bowl, toss the oil, sprouts, bacon, salt, and pepper.

3.  Place the sprouts on a rimmed baking sheet and bake, turning halfway through, for 20 minutes, or until the sprouts begin to brown.

4.  Divide the Brussels sprouts between 4 storage containers.

**Storage:** Place the airtight containers in the refrigerator for up to 5 days. You can freeze them, but the texture won't be great on thawing and reheating.

> **VARIATION TIP:** For added flavor, sprinkle with grated Parmesan cheese just before serving.

Per Serving: Calories: 347; Total Fat: 26g; Protein: 16g; Total Carbs: 16g; Net Carbs: 10g; Fiber: 6g; Sodium: 931mg

**Macros: 67% Fat; 18% Protein; 15% Carbs**

# CHEESY GREEN BEAN CASSEROLE

**MAKES 4 SERVINGS**

PREP TIME: 10 minutes    COOK TIME: 15 minutes

This is a great holiday side dish, but it's really delicious anytime of the year, even though it traditionally only comes out at the holidays. It makes use of two prep recipes already in this book, the Cream of Mushroom Soup (page 112) and the Caramelized Onions (page 130).

3 cups cooked green beans (fresh or frozen; if frozen, thaw them)

2 cups Cream of Mushroom Soup (page 112), cooled

½ cup Caramelized Onions (page 130)

½ cup shredded Cheddar cheese

1. Preheat the oven to 350°F.

2. In a large bowl, mix together the beans, soup, onions, and cheese.

3. Spread the mixture in a 9-by-13-inch baking dish and bake, uncovered, in the preheated oven until hot and bubbling, about 15 minutes.

4. Into each of 4 storage containers, place 1 cup of the casserole.

**Storage:** Place the airtight container in the refrigerator for up to 5 days. Reheat in the microwave 1 to 2 minutes or in a 350°F oven for about 15 minutes.

**COOKING TIP:** To cook fresh green beans, cut them in half lengthwise and snap off the stems. Cook in boiling water for about 4 minutes.

Per Serving: Calories: 366; Total Fat: 31g; Protein: 15g; Total Carbs: 18g; Net Carbs: 12g; Fiber: 6g; Sugar: 5g; Sodium: 403mg

**Macros: 76% Fat; 16% Protein; 8% Carbs**

# SPICY DEVILED EGGS

**MAKES 12 EGG HALVES**

PREP TIME: 10 minutes

These will keep for a few days in the refrigerator, and they travel well. They don't require any reheating, so they are perfect for picnics or quick work meals. Just carry them in a cooler with a little ice to keep them from spoiling when you take them with you.

6 Hard-boiled Eggs (page 82), peeled and halved lengthwise

½ cup Mayonnaise (page 87)

1 teaspoon Dijon mustard

1 dill pickle, minced

2 scallions, both white and green parts, minced

⅛ teaspoon cayenne pepper

1 garlic clove, minced

½ teaspoon salt

1. Scoop the yolks from the whites and put them in a small bowl. Place the whites, cut-side up, on a platter.

2. In the bowl, mix the yolks with the Mayonnaise, mustard, pickle, scallions, cayenne, garlic, and salt. Mix with a fork, mashing the egg yolks, until well combined.

3. Spoon or pipe into the egg white halves.

4. Into each of 6 storage containers, place 2 egg halves.

**Storage:** Place the airtight containers in the refrigerator for up to 5 days.

Per Serving (1 egg half): Calories: 72; Total Fat: 6g; Protein: 3g; Total Carbs: 3g; Net Carbs: 3g; Fiber <1g; Sodium: 249mg

**Macros: 75% Fat; 17% Protein; 8% Carbs**

# BAKED JALAPEÑO POPPERS

**MAKES 8 SERVINGS**

PREP TIME: 10 minutes    COOK TIME: 25 minutes

You may want to wear gloves when you prepare these to protect your skin from the oils in jalapeños, particularly if you have sensitive skin. These reheat especially well, so they make great meals or snacks on the go.

6 ounces cream cheese, at room temperature

½ cup shredded pepper Jack cheese, with a little reserved for garnish

16 jalapeño peppers, halved lengthwise with seeds and ribs removed

8 slices Perfectly Cooked Bacon (page 79), crumbled

1. Preheat the oven to 350°F.

2. In a bowl, combine the cream cheese and pepper Jack cheese.

3. Spoon the cheese mixture into the halved jalapeños and place them, cheese-side up, on a rimmed baking sheet. Sprinkle with the bacon and top with the cheese.

4. Bake until the cheese is melted and bubbling, about 25 minutes.

5. Into each of 8 storage containers, place 4 pepper halves.

**Storage:** Place the airtight containers in the refrigerator for up to 5 days. Reheat in the microwave for 1 to 2 minutes or in a 350°F oven for 15 to 20 minutes.

**VARIATION TIP:** Want it spicier? Add cayenne to the cream cheese mixture to your heat tolerance (remember, a little goes a long way). Want milder? Make sure all the seeds are removed from the jalapeños and replace the pepper Jack cheese with Cheddar.

Per Serving: Calories: 240; Total Fat: 20g; Protein: 12g; Total Carbs: 3g; Net Carbs: 3g; Fiber: <1g; Sodium: 592mg

**Macros: 76% Fat; 20% Protein; 4% Carbs**

# CREAM CHEESE AND CARAMELIZED ONION DIP WITH VEGGIES

**MAKES 6 SERVINGS**

PREP TIME: 10 minutes    COOK TIME: 20 minutes

If you have a batch of premade caramelized onions in your refrigerator or freezer, then you can make this dip very quickly. Allow the onions to cool almost completely before adding them to the dip.

¼ cup avocado oil

2 onions, sliced thinly, or ½ recipe Caramelized Onions (page 130)

1 teaspoon dried thyme

½ teaspoon salt

8 ounces cream cheese, at room temperature

¼ cup Mayonnaise (page 87)

1 teaspoon Dijon mustard

2 red bell peppers, sliced

1. In a large nonstick skillet, heat the oil over medium-high heat until it shimmers.

2. Reduce the heat to medium-low and add the onions, thyme, and salt.

3. Cook, stirring occasionally, until the onions are deeply caramelized, 20 to 30 minutes. Cool.

4. In a large bowl, combine the onions, cream cheese, Mayonnaise, and mustard. Mix until well combined.

5. Into each of 6 storage containers, divide the pepper strips, and into each of 6 separate storage containers, place ¼ cup dip.

**Storage:** Place the airtight containers in the refrigerator for up to 3 days. You can cook and freeze the onions ahead and thaw them to add into the dip, but don't freeze the dip.

**VARIATION TIP:** If you're looking for a little heat, add a few dashes of Tabasco sauce when you mix the dip together.

Per Serving: Calories: 211; Total Fat: 18g; Protein: 4g; Total Carbs: 10g; Net Carbs: 8g; Fiber: 2g; Sodium: 350mg

**Macros: 77% Fat; 8% Protein; 15% Carbs**

# SPINACH AND CHEESE STUFFED MUSHROOMS

**MAKES 8 SERVINGS**

PREP TIME: 10 minutes   COOK TIME: 25 minutes

While these make a delicious passed appetizer for parties, they're also super tasty as a meal or snack on the go. They taste good warm or cold, making them a great choice for when you don't have access to a microwave or oven.

8 ounces cream cheese, at room temperature

4 ounces frozen spinach, thawed, wrung dry, and chopped

1 teaspoon Dijon mustard

2 dashes Tabasco sauce

1 teaspoon garlic powder

1 tablespoon minced shallot

½ cup grated Parmesan cheese

1 pound button mushrooms, stemmed

1. Preheat the oven to 425°F.

2. In a large bowl, mix the cream cheese, spinach, mustard, Tabasco, garlic powder, shallot, and Parmesan.

3. Place the mushrooms on a rimmed baking sheet, cap-side down.

4. Spoon the filling generously into each mushroom cap.

5. Bake for 25 minutes. Let cool.

6. Divide the mushrooms between 8 storage containers.

**Storage:** Place the airtight containers in the refrigerator for up to 5 days. Reheat in the microwave for 1 or 2 minutes or in a 350°F oven for about 25 minutes.

**INGREDIENT TIP:** To clean mushrooms, wipe away any dirt with a damp paper towel. Don't run them under water, because they absorb water and will get spongy.

Per Serving: Calories: 162; Total Fat: 13g; Protein: 9g; Total Carbs: 4g; Net Carbs: 4g; Fiber: <1g; Sodium: 236mg

**Macros: 72% Fat; 22% Protein; 6% Carbs**

# COCONUT CHOCOLATE MOUSSE

**MAKES 6 SERVINGS**

PREP TIME: 10 minutes

Coconut cream makes a great base for a non-dairy dessert. To make coconut cream, place a can of full-fat coconut milk in the refrigerator overnight. The solids will rise to the top and the water will move to the bottom. Get rid of the water (or add it to thin to the desired consistency) and use just the cream.

2 (13.6-ounce) cans coconut milk, cream only, plus about ¼ cup coconut water, if needed, to thin to desired consistency

2 ounces unsweetened baking chocolate, melted and cooled slightly

1 teaspoon espresso powder

1 teaspoon liquid stevia or to taste

½ teaspoon vanilla extract

1. In a medium bowl, whisk together the coconut cream, chocolate, espresso powder, stevia, and vanilla until well combined.

2. Thin to the desired consistency with water from the coconut milk or with additional unseparated coconut milk.

3. Divide the mousse between 6 storage containers.

**Storage:** Place the airtight containers in the refrigerator for up to 5 days. You can also freeze this and cut it into squares to make fudge.

**VARIATION TIP:** Add up to a ½ cup of melted peanut butter and omit the espresso powder to make chocolate peanut butter mousse.

Per Serving: Calories: 396; Total Fat: 41g; Protein: 5g; Total Carbs: 11g; Net Carbs: 6g; Fiber: 5g; Sodium: 25mg

**Macros: 93% Fat; 5% Protein; 2% Carbs**

# BLENDED STRAWBERRY-COCONUT ICE POPS

**MAKES 4 SERVINGS**

PREP TIME: 10 minutes, plus overnight freezing

**Strawberries are one of the lowest-carb fruits, which makes them perfect for a quick keto snack. If you don't have ice pop molds, you can pour the mixture into paper cups, place foil over the top, and push a stick through the foil to freeze.**

1 cup halved strawberries

1 (13.6-ounce) can full-fat coconut milk

½ teaspoon liquid stevia

**1.** In a blender or food processor, combine the strawberries, coconut milk, and stevia. Blend until smooth.

**2.** Pour into ice pop molds and freeze overnight before serving.

**Storage:** Place the ice pops in the freezer for up to 6 months.

Per Serving: Calories: 272; Total Fat: 27g; Protein: 3g; Total Carbs: 9g; Net Carbs: 6g; Fiber: 3g; Sodium: 17mg

**Macros: 89% Fat; 4% Protein; 7% Carbs**

# CHOCOLATE-ALMOND FAT BOMBS

**MAKES 12 FAT BOMBS**

PREP TIME: 10 minutes, plus at least 1 hour chilling time

Fat bombs can help you adjust your macros if you haven't had enough fat to hit your daily goal. You can use candy molds, mini muffin tins, or even ice cube trays to make individual portions.

1 cup almond butter

2 ounces unsweetened baking chocolate

1 cup coconut oil

Liquid stevia

**1.** In a saucepan on low, combine the almond butter, chocolate, oil, and stevia to taste.

**2.** Cook, stirring, until melted and mixed. Taste to adjust the sweetness.

**3.** Pour into candy molds, ice cube trays, or mini muffin tins.

**4.** Chill for at least an hour. Pop out of the molds and transfer to a storage container.

**Storage:** Place the airtight container in the refrigerator for up to 5 days or freeze for up to 6 months.

Per Serving (1 fat bomb): Calories: 188; Total Fat: 21g; Protein: <1g; Total Carbs: 2g; Net Carbs: 2g; Fiber: <1g; Sodium: 1mg

**Macros: 99% Fat; <1% Protein; <1% Carbs**

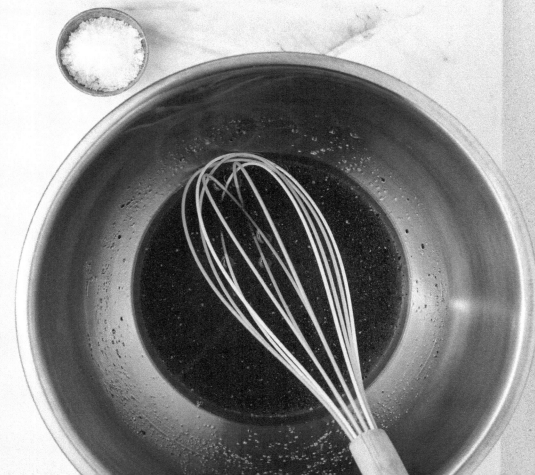

# Measurement Conversions

## Volume Equivalents (Liquid)

| US STANDARD | US STANDARD (OUNCES) | METRIC (APPROXIMATE) |
|---|---|---|
| 2 TABLESPOONS | 1 FL. OZ. | 30 ML |
| ¼ CUP | 2 FL. OZ. | 60 ML |
| ½ CUP | 4 FL. OZ. | 120 ML |
| 1 CUP | 8 FL. OZ. | 240 ML |
| 1½ CUPS | 12 FL. OZ. | 355 ML |
| 2 CUPS OR 1 PINT | 16 FL. OZ. | 475 ML |
| 4 CUPS OR 1 QUART | 32 FL. OZ. | 1 L |
| 1 GALLON | 128 FL. OZ. | 4 L |

## Volume Equivalents (Dry)

| US STANDARD | METRIC (APPROXIMATE) |
|---|---|
| ⅛ TEASPOON | 0.5 ML |
| ¼ TEASPOON | 1 ML |
| ½ TEASPOON | 2 ML |
| ¾ TEASPOON | 4 ML |
| 1 TEASPOON | 5 ML |
| 1 TABLESPOON | 15 ML |
| ¼ CUP | 59 ML |
| ⅓ CUP | 79 ML |
| ½ CUP | 118 ML |
| ⅔ CUP | 156 ML |
| ¾ CUP | 177 ML |
| 1 CUP | 235 ML |
| 2 CUPS OR 1 PINT | 475 ML |
| 3 CUPS | 700 ML |
| 4 CUPS OR 1 QUART | 1 L |
| ½ GALLON | 2 L |
| 1 GALLON | 4 L |

## Oven Temperatures

| FAHRENHEIT (F) | CELSIUS (C) (APPROXIMATE) |
|---|---|
| 250°F | 120°C |
| 300°F | 150°C |
| 325°F | 165°C |
| 350°F | 180°C |
| 375°F | 190°C |
| 400°F | 200°C |
| 425°F | 220°C |
| 450°F | 230°C |

## Weight Equivalents

| US STANDARD | METRIC (APPROXIMATE) |
|---|---|
| ½ OUNCE | 15 GRAMS |
| 1 OUNCE | 30 GRAMS |
| 2 OUNCES | 60 GRAMS |
| 4 OUNCES | 115 GRAMS |
| 8 OUNCES | 225 GRAMS |
| 12 OUNCES | 340 GRAMS |
| 16 OUNCES OR 1 POUND | 455 GRAMS |

# Recipe Index

# Index

# Acknowledgments

I'm genuinely grateful for the amount of support I received in creating and writing this cookbook. Without the love from my family and friends, it wouldn't have come together like it did. (Or at all for that matter!)

Thank you to my husband, Danny, for holding down the fort and doing more dishes than anyone ever should.

I want to thank my dad for his eclectic taste and passion for cooking. Watching his love in the kitchen is what led me to find my own passion for creating in the kitchen.

Thank you to my sweet mother, her creative gene, and her ability to create magical memories around the dinner table.

Thanks to my dearest friend, Laura, for believing in me since day one. Your drive is like nothing I've ever witnessed and has encouraged me to push past boundaries I didn't know I could.

Thanks to my Traeger family, especially Chad. Couldn't have done it without your support!

Thank you to Ms. Jocie and Ms. Holly for taking such good care of my Gracie Rose—I couldn't have done this without the two of you!

Thank you to the team at Callisto Media. So much went on behind the scenes, and they were so great to work with through this process.

Thanks to my family at 7K Fit—you have been so welcoming and supportive of my little family and our move to Evanston. Each of you inspire us on the daily and have made our dreams come true. That connection brought me the ketogenic online community, to whom I offer my greatest thanks. Without the support from my followers, Facebook group members, and the wonderful friends I have met, this opportunity simply would not have happened. Your stories, examples, and ketogenic transformations inspire me. Because of you I am passionate about sharing the tools, recipes, and inspiration that all of us can gain through living a ketogenic lifestyle.

Thank you to every one of you who provided encouragement, offered input, inspired the recipes, and brought this book to life.

To you the reader, I hope you discover the positive difference this can make in your life, and in the lives of those you love.

# About the Author

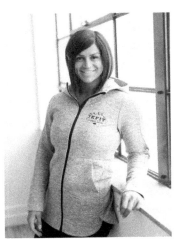

**Liz Williams** has devoted her career to helping others stay fit and feel good on the ketogenic diet. As part of her personal and professional commitment to health and wellness, she and her husband Danny operate the gym 7K Fit. Liz is also the author of *The One-Pot Ketogenic Diet Cookbook*. Follow her experiences with the ketogenic diet on her popular Instagram account @TheFitTrainersWife. Liz lives in Evanston, Wyoming, with her daughter and husband.

CPSIA information can be obtained
at www.ICGtesting.com
Printed in the USA
LVHW050154071118
596127LV00001BK/1

9 781641 522472